W9-CIP-471

Mr. Darrell Vollmar
8413 Peekskill Ln.
Houston, TX 77075-3013

Dian Dincin Buchman's

HERBAL
MEDICINE

Dian Dincin Buchman's

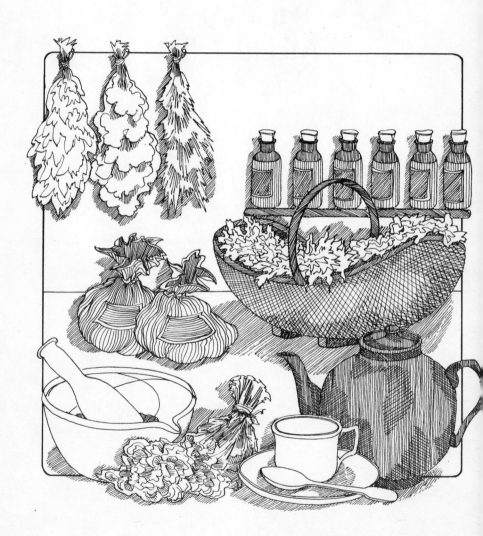

HERBAL MEDICINE

The Natural Way to

Get Well and Stay Well

Illustrated by Lauren Jarrett

David McKay Company, Inc.
NEW YORK

Library of Congress Cataloging in Publication Data

Buchman, Dian Dincin.
Dian Dincin Buchman's Herbal medicine.

Includes index.
1. Materia medica, Vegetable. 2. Herbs —Therapeutic
use. 3. Medicine—Formulae, receipts, prescriptions.
I. Title.   II. Title: Herbal medicine.
RS164.B78   615'.321   79-17005
ISBN 0-679-51080-X
ISBN 0-679-51081-8 pbk.

Book design by Linda Readerman

1 2 3 4 5 6 7 8 9 10

MANUFACTURED IN THE UNITED STATES OF AMERICA

For My Mother
Renee Dincin
and My Daughter
Caitlin Dincin Buchman

Important

Please refer to the Special Notice to the Reader on page *xx* and the instructions on page 117.

CONTENTS

Section Two: A Herbal Selector

Important

Please refer to the Special Notice to the Reader on page *xx* and the instructions on page 117.

PREFACE

In the not too distant past, many families had favorite home remedies. These were used to control small medical emergencies, and to prevent minor ailments from developing into chronic problems.

Naturally, every family had only snippets of home doctoring knowledge, but during this period there was also a considerable partnership between the home folks and the family doctor, and physicians often used a variety of plant and water remedies to cure common ills. Indeed, until the 1940s textbooks of pharmacognosy—books that relate the use of plants for proven prescription medicine—contained hundreds of useful comments on barks, roots, berries, leaves, resins, twigs, and flowers.

In my own family, different people were the keepers of various recipes. An aunt knew how to make a bruise ointment, an uncle a tonic rosemary wine, and my grandmother made and taught us how to make cold creams, vinegars and poultices. These handed-down tonics, ointments, and liniments, our European "secret" remedies, were developed through generations of observation in home care.

However, as twentieth-century technology advanced, and there came into being a constant and upward spiral of admiration for technology and technologists, most simple plant and water therapy remedies were declared useless, and gradually discarded. The past was dead; only new things could possibly work, went the litany. Suddenly, self-sufficient people felt only the fruits of new science were appropriate for medical care. The family relinquished its memories of home first aid, and banished home control of even minor health problems.

This unconscious and gradual cultural withdrawal had many serious consequences. Although there was no awareness of the process, large groups of people became more and more alienated from their ethnic roots and lost their sense of self-sufficiency and hence lost a great deal of self-esteem. This lowering of self-esteem coincided with the feeling that no one had control over his or her own body, which in turn led to an increase in passivity and a feeling of helplessness.

Recent studies indicate that people who feel helpless may contract a serious chronic disease as a result, and sometimes do not recover their health precisely because they perceive themselves as totally helpless.

Thus life-saving technology produced a more dependent, less self-sufficient person. Old health concepts based on simple and useful observations vanished. People were ashamed to talk about the value of sunshine, about walking outdoors to feel better, about how the best two doctors are the right foot and left foot, about breathing deeply to eliminate stress, "sweating it out," about spring cures (body cleansing after long, hard winters). Rough, chewy, "old fashioned" food was rejected, and devitalized white bread, as delicious as library paste, took its place along with soft foods, hormone-injected meat, and chemicalized fruits and vegetables. Alas, the number of chemicals added to food is now so large, that it is said a Thanksgiving meal will provide a thousand chemicals. My friend, Beatrice Trum Hunter, describes this state of events as "the great nutrition robbery."

Although people are living longer, they are not necessarily feeling better, and there has been a vast interest in exercise programs, water as therapy, and drugless home doctoring. People are rediscovering their strong ethnic roots and rein-vestigating old values.

Now that the pendulum has started to swing there is even a danger that everything old will be considered of more value than anything new. I don't hold with the extremists of either side, and I feel I must pick the best of scientific knowledge as well as the most effective remedies of the past.

While herbs can act in an almost magical and astonishing way—spasms may relax, diarrhea vanish, constipation be overcome, nervousness recede, headaches disappear, colds be banished, blood flow be arrested—they do not answer *every* medical problem. It is still necessary to get routine medical checkups once in a while, and to have a good family doctor to consult in case of a health crisis.

Even so, you must try to become less passive, less like an "object" to be taken in a shopping bag to the doctor. And some people do think of themselves as a sort of a package they can deposit on the doctor's desk: "Here Doc, take this, and see what you can do."—almost the way you take a radio or a car in to be fixed.

You need to know about the forty nutrients the body needs each day to stay healthy, about your own exercise needs, how breathing can release stress and tension, and how water can relax, stimulate and relieve you. You will certainly know after reading this book how a few hundred everyday foods, spices, herbs, and some few special wild and garden herbs can be used to help you prevent or control many common health problems.

If you are new to the use of herbs for personal health, you will have to start a new regime of thinking like a herbalist. That means approaching each problem in a holistic way. You are a thinking being who can make his or her own appropriate judgments for everyday life and a person in partnership with a family physician.

A holistic approach means you will not list only the symptoms, but you will try to unearth the *causes* of the symptoms. Sometimes the cause will be obvious, and you can immediately alleviate or eliminate the causal factors. Other times the reasons for a symptom will be hidden, but since you will be thinking about it, an idea may pop out to redirect your activities. An example of this thinking might be working out the cause of a specific headache. Is the headache from a toothache? If you rub under the tooth, on the gum, and the headache goes away, you know you have a dental problem. In the meantime, if a dentist isn't immediately available, you can use the herbal therapy suggested here. If the headache is from eye strain, you can use pressure therapy over the optic nerves, and/or pads soaked in such herbs as witch hazel extract. That can encourage you to do strengthening eye exercises, and to get an eye checkup. Is the headache from tight shoes? Take a hot mustard foot bath—and change those shoes. Is the headache from indigestion? Try a digestive tea—there are loads of them in the book. In other words, be a detective. It's amazing how many problems you will solve for yourself. But if the headache persists, see a physician in any case.

Herbs can act differently on different people, and can also vary in strength from garden to garden, and lose strength from the way they are dried or stored; therefore, it is imperative that you buy your botanical health substances from the most reliable sources.

Remember: Herbal health care is only one of several systems, and you mustn't think these humble herbs can answer every single health problem. In this book I share my own herbal experience with you, but you must guard against putting blind faith in *any* panacea.

I suggest you capture and use only *one herb at a time*. In this way you will get clear in your mind the various ways each herb works. Then go on to another herb and conquer it, and practice with it. When you use only one herb at a time, it is called a "simple." Enjoy and use your herbal simples!

Dian Dincin Buchman

INTRODUCTION

Why We Should Use Herbal Medicine

Since early Neanderthal man, plants have been used for healing purposes. Even as modes of medicine changed throughout the centuries, plants continued to be the mainstay of country medicine as methods and ideas on plant healing were passed down from family to family, and within communities. Thus tribes, clans, villages, towns, sometimes entire countries, tended to have similar styles in healing. Most of these plant remedies were based on local discoveries and pass-along uses, so it is always interesting to note how many plants are used in exactly the same way. Chamomile, for instance, is a digestive aid throughout the world.

Even though much of the medical community ignores, perhaps even disdains, plant medicine as too old fashioned, plants are nontheless the basis for some of the most effective drugs. For several thousand years the Chinese physicians used the Ma Huang plant. Later researchers extracted an alkaloid, ephedrine, from this plant. This is still used in many different ways, namely for relief of nasal congestion, bronchial coughs and asthma. Unbeknown to the general public, pharmaceutical firms continue to comb the more primitive places on earth to explore and define native folk medicine. They bring back various botanical specimens in the hope of discovering plants that can be successfully duplicated.

An interesting example of this continuous interest in new products, and why some investigations are quickly discontinued, was described to me by Dr. Vera Stecher, an international pharmaceutical researcher. When her work brought her to Malawi, Africa, Dr. Stecher met a Dutch scientist, a recent victim of a painful and reccuring skin cancer. Although the cancer had been surgically removed several times in Switzerland, it always re-emerged on his hand. One day this Dutchman took a long motor ride to the interior of Malawi, and there on a dusty road he gave a ride to a hitchhiking old tribesman. That simple act was a happy turning point in his life. The dignified African soon observed his host's pain in clutching the steering wheel. With a sign he motioned the Dutchman to stop the jeep. The African then climbed out and quickly cut a large fruit from a common native tree.

With deft fingers, the tribal doctor applied the pulp of this fruit to the Dutchman's throbbing, aching hands. Within minutes the pain disappeared. Subsequent applications of this fresh pulp not only controlled all pain, but eventually eliminated the entire skin cancer! This same treatment also proved effective for several other Europeans who had similar skin cancers.

Dr. Stecher was naturally excited by her colleague's personal discovery. She carried large, whole fruits with her to Switzerland, her home laboratory base. The first results were outstanding. In the initial studies conducted by friends of Dr. Stecher, they found the fruit pulp did indeed control the artificially induced skin cancers of laboratory animals. Unfortunately, they did not get the same results when the fruit was chemically reproduced, and all future experiments were called off. Some plants cannot be successfully duplicated, and some plants, it seems, must be used only in the raw, fresh state.

Willow bark, one of nature's great anti-inflammatory plants, was used for thousands of years, even by American Indian tribes. Unfortunately, consistent use of the bark affected the digestive system, and it became imperative to find a substitute, or a chemical version. This duplication took over fifty years of investigation, and was solved when a clever German scientist broke the chemical code by using the spirea plant family, instead of willow bark. He called his result *aspirin*, now one of the most used drugs on earth.

History is studded with fascinating plant discoveries from primitive cultures, and some of these discoveries have even changed history and medicine. Ipecac, now used in the home as an emetic to disgorge poisons, once helped to control the savage dysentery that pervaded Europe. Quinine, from the tropics, saved the world from the ravages of malaria. Curare arrow poison, another tropical discovery, is now used to control breathing during some surgery.

My favorite plant story concerns a little old "herb lady" and William Withering, a curious and careful English country doctor, working during the eighteenth century. Dr. Withering was constantly aware of the limitations of his medical knowledge, and unceasing in his efforts to be a better doctor. Sadly he often sent his badly damaged heart patients home to die. "There is nothing more I can do for you." To his astonishment he would sometimes meet these same patients at local fairs. They were not only still alive, but hale and hearty. He finally asked some of them how they had achieved this miracle of life. To a man they had quaffed the bitter remedies of a plant lady, a strange, old woman who had the cure for dropsy, the fluid accumulation from heart, liver and kidney malfunction. Withering sought her out and she showed him her plant concoctions. Withering, an amateur botanist, instantly comprehended that the strongest of her plants was foxglove. He toiled ten years to isolate the active ingredient in this plant, and discovered digitalis, a substance still used in todays heart-saving medicine.

For centuries tribal doctors in Africa, and non-Western physicians in India, used preparations of the rauwolfia root to cure "moon madness." But this use for mental illness was ignored by all Western investigators until a certain incident occured in London. A young Nigerian prince, a student at a great English university, had a mental breakdown, and like Humpty Dumpty, none of the King's officers or men could put him back together again. Since no one could alleviate his distress, his fellow Nigerian students sent for a tribal doctor. He arrived with a batch of rauwolfia, and soon the young student was functioning in a normal way. The amazed British physicians instituted a major laboratory investigation of this root. The result—the first synthetic tranquilizer: reserpine, a breakthrough in working with the mentally ill. Reserpine is the base of about a dozen anti-hypertensive drugs which also sedate and tranquilize.

There are hundreds of such stories and many anecdotes of profound cures from either herbal simples (one vegetable substance) or herbal combinations. Many of these stories are lost forever, but only recently, as I discussed the rare virtues of the ginger root with my class at a local college, my student, Shirley Holmes, recalled that she had been saved from infant death by this plant.

Shirley had been born prematurely and was so small she couldn't be fed, and the doctor felt she couldn't live. Her Scottish grandmother asked if she could take the baby home as she was determined to give her ginger tea to survive. But the baby wouldn't drink the tea. The grandmother then hit on the marvelous notion of making a tea out of ginger snap cookies. The baby liked this ginger-tasting tea, and in three months, all was well.

Plants are effective medicine, but they aren't the only answer to good health. I urge you to a full investigation of these varied herbal simples and combinations, as *part* of your approach to holistic health practices. You should be striving to rebalance the body, to restore your native energy level so that the body can cure itself. Sometimes plants can achieve this rebalancing and internal cleansing of the body. Often a combination of water therapy and plants and nutrition is effective. Other times you might need pressure or manipulation techniques. With plants, and with water, you will have a considerable personal and natural home medicine chest for preventive health measures, first aid, and normal everyday health needs.

Many of the herbs presented in this book are foods that are in your refrigerator, or on your kitchen shelf. Some are also slightly more esoteric flowers, plants, leaves, barks, berries or roots. Many of these plants can be grown by you in your own backyards, and some will respond to window-sill gardening.

As far as I know, all these plants are available from responsible botanical firms, special pharmacies, or health stores. I have starred the firms that I know personally. Others I offer as resources in order that you may expand your local or mail-order contacts.

I give both detailed and brief vignettes of many useful medicinal herbs and foods. I urge you always to use herbs and plants in moderation even though they may be known to be safe for thousands of years. In prior centuries people mostly used local plants. We now use plants from all over the world. We do not always know how plants are picked, how dried. It is therefore important *to know your sources* for the plants you use. Let us hope for more and more organic (non-sprayed) sources.

This book can be used by novice herbalists, and I have deliberately ignored, or mention cautions on, those herbs that may be difficult or dangerous to use, especially if you are an inexperienced herbalist. In addition to the easy-to-follow directions throughout the book, there is *A Herbal Selector*, a section devoted to the herbal simples or combinations that are known to be helpful in minor health problems.

In some ways this is a personal home pharmacy workbook showing how plant chemicals are released for home use. The book describes step by step home preparations of infusions, tea blends, decoctions, tinctures, medicated wines, syrups, ointments, repellents, liniments, gargles, suppositorites, pills, lozenges, deodorants, poultices and various herbs for special use as compresses, packs and bath. This last subject is described in detail in *The Complete Book of Water Therapy*. Cosmetic and body care are fully described in *The Complete Herbal Guide To Natural Health and Beauty*.

SPECIAL NOTICE TO THE READER

The simple herbal palliatives in this book, using common herbs, must not be used as substitutes for professional medical attention for any serious health disturbance or for any chronic warning symptoms. When in doubt, consult your physician.

Some herbs may cause slightly undesirable side effects in some users. Therefore, try only one herb at a time and begin using that herb in small doses, experimentally, and wait and watch for such a side effect. If there is none, increase the use or the dosage cautiously and continue checking for reactions each time.

Not all herbal applications are effective in every case for every person. Nor does every person react the same way to the same herb. The user of herbs should therefore avoid drawing generalized conclusions from his or her use of an herb or from others' use.

The symbol ★ in conjunction with certain herbs throughout the book indicates that each such herb is to be considered for *preventive* use; that is, not just as a palliative for an existing ailment, but as an herb to be used regularly to prevent or make less likely the onset of the indicated ailment.

SECTION ONE

MY FAVORITE HERBS

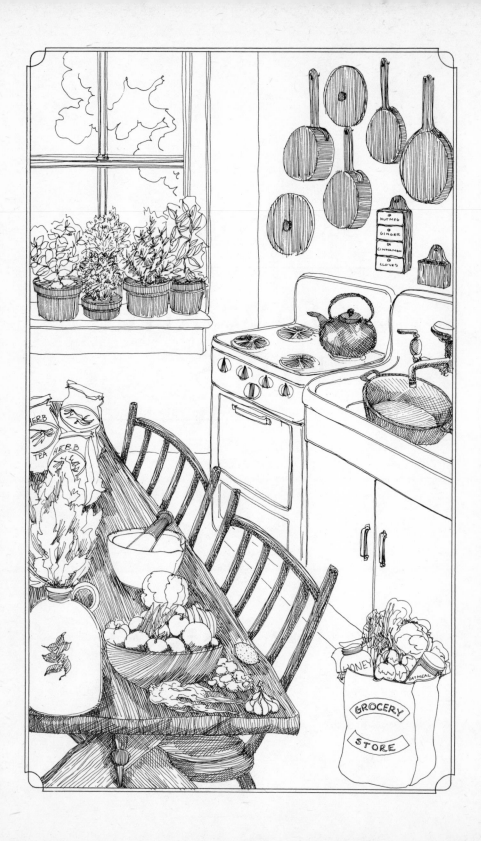

COMFREY
(Symphytum officinale)

Bonesetting   I have a friend who until recently was a leading executive employed by the Ford Foundation in India. He has told me many stories of Indian medicine, and he never ceased to be amazed at the unique "sect" of Indian bonesetters who heal their patients with secret plant preparations, manual setting of fractures, and no cast.

"What is so unusual," says my friend, "is that the patients—and my own son was one, and so was an eighty-year-old missionary woman friend—heal in a fraction of the time it takes with Western medicine!"

He says these bonesetting groups are dying out because they refuse to tell their age-old secrets to anyone outside their own families. One of the substances in their healing salve sounds as if it might be one of my favorite healing herbs, comfrey, which some English herbalists consider to be the most powerful healing agent in the plant world. This plant is not only available in live plant and seed form from many organic farmers in the United States, but it is also readily available in dried root, root powder, and leaf tea form from botanical sources or health-food stores.

Even if comfrey were not part of the Indian bonesetters' secret ointment, I would want to share with you the incredible virtues of this green plant. For medical purposes, mainly the root is used, but the leaf has excellent healing powers, too.

Ointment   I always try to have a comfrey *ointment* and a comfrey *tincture* in our nondrug medicine chest.

3

The ointment, which you can either make or buy in a health-food store or homeopathic pharmacy, I have used in innumerable first-aid cases for the family and visitors. Comfrey root ointment is really healing for almost any kind of sore or bruise or abrasion and, according to many ancient herbal healers, is effective for bones that grind and fracture—but I cannot personally attest to these last attributes.

Recently we had a physician and his wife as overnight guests, and although we have been friends for a long time, he believes in his form of medicine and I mine, so I was surprised when he said, "How about one of your special herbs for this sore around my lip?" I thought he was kidding me, but I did bring him some comfrey ointment, and he dabbed it around his mouth and on the sore.

The next morning he was most enthusiastic about the effect and insisted on taking some with him, as the sore had almost disappeared and he was convinced one more application would help. Weeks later he said it had been effective. Moreover he reported his teen-age son had also used it and had declared it "magic."

That's just about how the former generations of English countryfolk felt about comfrey symphytum. They called it by other names—knitbone, or bruisewort, names which describe its uses. Their praise for comfrey is high. In an old recipe book of a famout noble English family, I found this reference: "It is an *infallible* remedy for bruises, wounds, ruptures and hemorrhoids and even ulcers in the stomach."

Root   And what does the English herbalist Nicholas Culpeper say? His description is mind-boggling. He describes how he puts *bruised* comfrey roots "outwardly" on fresh wounds and cuts and then adds, "It is specially good for ruptures and broken bones, *so powerful to consolidate and knit together, that if they be boiled with dissevered pieces of flesh in a pot, it will join them together.*"

Indeed this root will produce a high amount of gummy substance, which herbalists call mucilage, and the root and the leaf are both high in allantoin, a substance that helps with cell proliferation. Mrs. M. Grieve, in *A Modern Herbal,* has conjectured that the healing ability of the plant is probably the result of the allantoin, and this may be the reason comfrey can reduce the swollen skin in the area of fractures, "causing the union to take place with greater facility."

The herbalist John Gerard also confirms this healing ability of comfrey, saying that in his experience, "A salve concocted from the fresh herb will certainly tend to promote the healing of bruised and broken parts."

Tincture Our family had an interesting experience with the tincture of comfrey. A tincture is a preparation of an herb soaked in alcohol or spirits of wine for enough time to absorb the principal chemicals of the plant. The plant is then strained away. (See "Tincture," Section Three.)

Working in our garden, my husband accidentally dropped a huge rock on his right big toe. The pain was excruciating and the bruise looked bad. Fortunately, I had some tinctures up at the cottage, and I immediately dropped about 15–20 drops of comfrey tincture in a pan of cold water for a half-hour foot soak. I also kept the toe soaked in wet dressings of diluted comfrey tincture that whole day and evening. I occasionally added some tincture of calendula.

Not realizing what a great pain he was avoiding thanks to the treatment, my husband kept on saying, "What's all the fuss? The foot doesn't hurt at all!"

I am delighted to report that he felt no further pain. The toe did look a sickly yellow-blue, but to our amazement, the nail stayed intact. And then after a time (it might have been a month or more—it was so very painless that no notice was taken of it) the nail fell off. Lo, there was a whole new nail underneath, though it did have some odd ridges, possibly as a result of the accident.

Friends who have had this kind of traumatic injury to their feet were just amazed at the fact that my husband had no pain and that the nail gave him no trouble. One of our neighbors told him, "I'll never forget the night a big heavy metal table fell on my foot, particularly the big toe. I had

incredible pain that first night—couldn't walk at all and I had
to stay in bed the next day—and I was in a terrible temper for
at least a week. Also,"—and she shook her head at the quick
recovery my husband had made—"I remember having foot
pain and trouble for at least six months afterward."

One of my favorite comfrey stories concerns an 18th
century journalist named Thompson. He had a terrible accident in the woods and was so badly wounded that his friends
and a local doctor wanted to take off his leg. He was almost
ready to let them do that when he decided to try comfrey
poultices on the chance it would help. Poultices of the root did
save his leg.

Then there is a fairly well-authenticated story of a locksman (a canal worker) in Teddington, England. The bone of his
little finger was broken and was grinding and "grunching" for
two long months. He was very uncomfortable, so one day he
spoke to a doctor travelling on the canal. The doctor smiled
and pointed to a huge green comfrey plant growing along the
canal path. "Take some of that root, wash it, chomp on it, and
put it around your finger and wrap it up," he said. Four days
later, as the doctor was making a return trip, the locksman was
happy to report, "I'm just fine now, doctor. My finger is well."
But we are talking of course about an era when common
wayside and garden plants were used daily for healing of
various problems.

Poultice   I like using comfrey root in various oils or lanolin to
produce a marvelous and healing ointment. I also use drops of
the comfrey tincture in water for various compresses.

The green leaves are slightly hairy, have a slightly sticky
surface and may be somewhat irritating on sensitive skin.
However comfrey poultices have been successful on insect
bites and burns.

Internal Use   Comfrey has so many healing properties that it
has long been used for its soothing and internally healing
qualities. It contains a great deal of B_{12} a vitamin hard to find in
other plants, and has long been used as a source of this
vitamin, particularly by vegans.

Because comfrey can heal the digestive tract, it is also often combined with pepsin or fenugreek in tablet form, or powder form for internal use.

It now appears that this use of comfrey may not be safe. The latest laboratory research has uncovered alarming news about the internal use of *young* comfrey leaves. The news is the result of work done by the prestigious Henry Doubleday Research Association of Great Britain, an organization devoted to organic farming, and the use of comfrey as a world food. Since this organization has been in the forefront of the interest in comfrey, its suggestions and facts and bulletins must be taken very seriously. They report the following:

Comfrey is in the same plant family as several other plants (Senecio, Crotolaria, Heliotropium), and these plants, investigation now indicates, contain some natural poisons in the form of *pyrrolizidine alkaloids*. These plants have been implicated in various accidental human and animal poisonings.

The young leaves of comfrey, thought to be so edible and rich in chlorophyll, and used in many natural green drinks, may contain up to 0.15 percent (1,500 parts per million) of the alkaloid.

Dr. Claude Culvenor of the Animal Health Division of the Australian Commonwealth Scientific and Industrial Research Organization has worked on this subject and studied this alkaloid in pasture weeds. He is particularly conversant with heliotrope, a weed from the same plant family as comfrey.

He notes "At least four of these alkaloids are known to be carcinogens, and it is probable that the type found in comfrey is also carcinogenic. While it is unlikely that anybody eating comfrey in small quantities would suffer serious effects, its regular use as a green vegetable could cause chronic liver damage or worse.

"Plants in the same family have caused human poisonings in the USSR, Africa, India and Afghanistan after their accidental consumption in bread over a period of one or two years.

"The evidence of these outbreaks, considering the amount of the alkaloid we have measured in comfrey, suggests that daily consumption of several young leaves of the plant over a similarly lengthy period will lead to serious disease."

According to an interesting article in the New York State Natural Foods Associates Newsletter which led me to the information contained in this caution, it has been suggested that there may be some hidden factor in comfrey which protects against these alkaloids, since it has been fed with seeming immunity to racehorses, and livestock throughout the world.

The Henry Doubleday Research Association is continuing its research on comfrey, and it may well find there is some compensating factor in comfrey which cancels out the alkaloid. While the organization believes that comfrey *ointment*, which shows only 3 parts per million of the alkaloid, is *entirely safe* for *external use*, and the fresh leaves, pulped leaves, or comfrey flour is safe to use as *poultices*, it indicates that until additional research is available, human beings *should not eat or drink comfrey in any form.*

Powder   Comfrey also comes in powder form. "Use it dry or as a wet mash on troublesome growths and oversize persistent body warts," says Dr. Kirschner in *Nature's Healing Grasses.*

To use the root powder, dampen it with water until it forms a gummy mass. Place this mass in a clean handkerchief and apply it to bruises, inflammations, ulcers, and sores.

On the whole, comfrey is easier to use in ointment form, unless you have large areas to heal, and here the root or the leaf poultices would be easier and cheaper to use.

Arthritis   Swiss physician Alfred Vogel says to apply softened comfrey roots to alleviate pain of arthritis. "The pain will gradually fade out," according to him. Dr. Vogel, author of *The Nature Doctor*, also uses comfrey for gout as well as for broken bones.

CHAMOMILE
(Anthemis nobilis)

This is one of the most versatile and benign of all the herbs and has been used for hundreds, perhaps thousands, of years all over the world. My grandmother was particularly fond of chamomile flowers, and she always had a huge jar of them in her house. When someone seemed ill, her hand would plunge into the bell-shaped chamomile jar she kept in the kitchen, and she would make a "tisane," a tea. Before long, the person would start to feel more relaxed. She felt that chamomile, while quite sedative and quieting, was also a tonic, and she always made the grandchildren use it when we were irritable.

Digestion ★ Chamomile is a wonder herb for digestion, weak stomach, stomach spasms, and for anything related to digestion. Prepare the flowers in tea form, one to two tablespoons to a cup of boiling water. Drink half a cupful at a time.

Stomachache Chamomile is soothing and sedative for the body, especially for a tummy-ache. There is an old tradition in Europe for mothers to use a weak chamomile tea, or a linden (lime-blossom tea, called "tilia" in France), to calm a tormented teething baby or to help overcome colic spasms. As a young mother I often made such a weak brew of chamomile for my daughter to alleviate any digestive distress. Strain before adding it to the bottle, and use in diluted form. Make sure your dried chamomile (a ground cover) contains no ragweed.

Diarrhea Chamomile is an old remedy for children's summer diarrhea.

Nightmare ★ I owe my great interest in herbal lore to my grandmother, who learned some of her remedies and attitudes from gypsies who lived or wandered near her remote Rumanian border village. When grandmother's innkeeper-father died, these gypsies escorted her across Rumania to her father's people. These gypsies believed chamomile was a preventive for nightmares, and thus on a thundery night or on a day awash in stress, she always persuaded us to "drink the cham."

Old Age Tea On the opposite side of the age seesaw, old

people revere chamomile as a helpful tea. Buy some for your favorite grandmother or grandfather, and also use some for yourself; chamomile tea is used all over the world as a table tea. For older people and young children, the tea, drunk one hour before dinner, is said to sharpen dull appetites, and is also calming and pleasant as well as slightly stimulating. Use thirty flowers to a jug of boiling water. Steep for fifteen minutes and strain.

Allergy to Chamomile? Chamomile flowers are low growing and are sometimes incorrectly picked with some ragweed content. If you are allergic to ragweed, be very certain of your chamomile source. Dr. Walter Lewis of Washington University in St. Louis, Missouri, has suggested in interviews that ragweed content may influence allergic response in some people.

Enema Chamomile tea may be used to irrigate the body when there are chronic stomach spasms caused by gas. This and a neutral, natural, and fibre-rich diet will often cure the flatulence.

I once had an interesting call from an older woman, a friend of the family and the widow of a physician. She was trying to recapture her health without drugs and told me she was tired of working only on symptoms, hoping instead to attack the causes. She was trying to recall the wonderful stomach herb of her childhood and was delighted when I asked if she meant chamomile.

She drank chamomile tea, took chamomile enemas, started to eat fibrous vegetables, fruit, and oatmeal, and soon called to say the gas pains had disappeared. At my suggestion she also continued this regime along with vigorous hand and foot massage.

Antiseptic, Antipain Chamomile is said to be more antiseptic than seawater. The herbalist Parkinson has written, "Chamomile is put to divers and sundry uses, both for pleasure and profit, both for the sick and the sound, in bathing to comfort and strengthen the sound, and to ease pain in the diseased."

To attempt to reduce inflammation, sores and swellings, apply the chamomile hot and wet in a paste. To make paste, add a small amount of boiling water to the flowers, and blend in a blender or grind together in a mortar and pestle.

Bath and Hair   Make up a large infusion, steep for fifteen minutes, strain, and add to a bath to heal body sores and aches. "Bathing with chamomile removes weariness and eases pain to whatever part of the body it is employed," says Culpeper.

This same infusion can be used to lighten and add golden highlights to mousey brown hair. Chamomile combines well with neutral henna, too, to add beautiful highlights to dark hair.

Facials   Georgette Klinger runs a fine European-style facial salon on Madison Avenue in New York and another in Beverly Hills, California. She tells me that chamomile facials are "penetrating." The deep pore-cleansing given at this salon includes a chamomile facial. Boil water, add it to chamomile flowers, and improvise an umbrella "hood" with a large towel. Keep your eyes closed and allow the chamomile steam to open the pores of your face. This will help to release embedded dirt and blackheads. Be careful to stay out of a draft and to cleanse your face immediately after the facial.

Insect Repellent ★   With the tea splashed over my face, arms, hands, and feet, mosquitoes won't come near me. The sweet, apple-like smell is also usually repugnant to gnats and summer flies.

Chamomile should be a staple in your herbal cupboard. It can be obtained in flower, tea bag, tincture, extract, and fresh organic juice form.

BERRIES

Blackberry *(Rubus fructicosus)*

As I am about to write the words "berries are herbs," a strange panorama stirs across my mind and I am returned to a vignette of childhood. I remember my mother asking me to walk down the road from our Long Pond summer cottage to pick some blackberries, although I often ate more than I brought back home. Of course, we usually used these berries for dessert, but on occasion I recall my mother saying, "This batch is for the vinegar," or "this batch is for the powder." Both were extraordinarily effective medicines.

Diarrhea ★   The powder that I am speaking of was made from fresh whole, dried blackberries. After washing them, mother dried and heated them in the sun or in a moderately hot oven until the berries were dry and could be powdered. This powder was put away in a tightly shut jar labeled "D." I somehow thought the "D" meant Dincin, but when I was about six I learned it actually meant diarrhea. Blackberries in all forms are a resource against the runs!

In addition to this marvelous storable powder which can be stored away, fresh blackberries, blackberry bark, blackberry leaves, and even blackberry root are effective herbal medicine for what those old herbalists called "relaxed bowels." The powder is taken in teaspoon doses with a small amount of water, but tea made from the leaves (pour boiling water over the leaves and steep them for five minutes) or the water from the simmered bark or root can be used in cup doses several times a day. In addition you can use the fresh blackberries when on a backpacking trip. You can obtain blackberry leaves from many health-food stores, or you can dry your own.

Cordial—Restorative ★   The *London Pharmacopoeia of 1679* describes ripe blackberries as an excellent cordial and restorative. That means you can use blackberries to stimulate the body and the heart, and they can be used to good effect in overcoming an illness. A blackberry extract or concentrated blackberry juice is sometimes available in health-food stores. Add a dash to any herbal tea such as chamomile or peppermint, for a lift, to cleanse the body of impurities.

Ulcers I found another blackberry cure in Cruso's 1771 *Treasury of Easy Medicine,* which I read in a British library. Here the author advises soaking blackberry leaves in a hot wine infusion and placing the hot leaves on ulcers every morning and evening. "Which will heal them, however difficult to be cured," he says.

Gargle The Cruso wine infusion would also be a fine gargle for a sore throat, but then *any* blackberry preparation helps with sore throat. We often use blackberry jelly added to a hot peppermint leaf tea for an instant gargle. We also use raspberry vinegar compresses on the throat. To do this, dip a cloth into the vinegar, wring it out, and wind it around the throat. Add a layer or two of dry cloths, or attach an old woolen sock. This helps relax the throat.

I should mention, too, that apple cider vinegar also works as a gargle and a sore throat aid and can be used in the very same way.

Swelling Blackberry jelly was also used by the country people of England for swelling of the limbs, particularly the kind that comes as a result of heart trouble. To use, add the jelly to apple cider vinegar and apply it as a compress.

We used to make a stimulating blackberry cordial and a vinegar which seemed to meet many physical problems with quick and ready help.

Blackberry Cordial To make this cordial, gather fresh blackberries and press out the juice. For every quart of this juice, add ½ ounce each of nutmeg and cloves and 2 pounds of sugar, or slightly less honey. Simmer these together for a short time until everything looks syrupy. Cool it and add brandy to taste.

A word about sugar. When used to excess it is a destructive substance. I now use a good uncooked honey for these and other recipes. While it is hard to be accurate about the replacement of honey in recipes, I usually replace with an equal weight of sugar to light honey. This works out to ⅔ of a cup of liquefied honey to 1 cup of dry sugar. However, in general, remember that you also have to deduct 3 tablespoons of any other liquid from the recipe for each cup of honey you use. If the honey gets stiff, warm it up with a little warm water first. Unfortunately, honey syrup does not keep as well as the sugar syrup, and it may ferment if unrefrigerated. (See "Honey—Cooking With.")

Blackberry Vinegar ★ This vinegar mixed with water will quench the thirst when all other beverages have failed.

It can be given to patients with fever.

It is a cordial for those who have a cold with fever.

The ancient herbals state that when you add this vinegar to distilled water, the combination eases and dissolves the deposits of gout and arthritis.

Gather the berries and take them off the stalks. Place the berries in malt or apple cider vinegar in a covered ceramic, stainless, cast iron, nonaluminum pot. Let the mixture stand for three days to draw the berry juices into the vinegar, then allow the berries to drip all day through a strainer. Measure the juice. Add about a pound of honey for each pint of juice. Simmer gently for five minutes or so. Remove any scum as it appears, then set the blackberry vinegar aside to cool. Bottle and label it correctly and close it with a tight lid or cork. (Note my comments under Red Raspberry for a shortcut.)

Blackberry Glycerite This compound is another blackberry medicinal. You make this in the same way as vinegar, except that instead of adding honey to the strained blackberry vinegar juice, you add 8 ounces of glycerine to each pint of juice. Boil this together and skim. When it is cool, bottle and label it and keep it in a cool place. Glycerine is an excellent preservative.

Both the vinegar and the glycerite can be used as external compresses on swollen arthritic joints.

Red Raspberry

The red raspberry can be used in many of the same ways as the blackberry. It, too, may be effective with sore throat, especially one associated with a bad cold or flu. And a drink of red raspberry vinegar and water will also bring down a fever.

Vinegar   There is a shortcut in making either blackberry or red raspberry vinegar. Add hot vinegar to a raspberry jelly, or to syrup. Blackberry or raspberry syrup can help you to dissolve the tartar on your teeth. But the mouth must be rinsed immediately, as this mixture has a high sugar content.

Mouth Blisters   Raspberry or blackberry shoots may be boiled in water and the cooled water rinsed through the mouth to reduce mouth blisters.

Woman's Herb ★   Red raspberry leaf is an important woman's herb. An experienced midwife told me she always used red raspberry leaf tea to reduce bleeding during childbirth. She also suggests it for morning sickness and during delivery. Patients are to use it warm and in huge quantities. Red raspberry tea also can help where there is a too-profuse menstrual flow. It is soothing and nonstimulating and can slowly decrease the flow. Combine it with cinnamon bark or cinnamon powder.

ARNICA
(Arnica montana)

Reflections

As I look back on my childhood, I realize that our household was considered an unmodern one by our neighbors, friends, and some relatives. My parents disdained

drugstore first aid. Our "medicine chest" had home ointments, tinctures, liniments, and gargles made from *plants*. Of
course we children resisted this old-fashioned concept sometimes, as we preferred to be "modern" just like everyone else.

But when I think of childhood and the gentle ministration
of my mother when I had pain from falls, strains, or unbroken
bruises, it brings to mind the remarkable plant arnica.

Ancestral Uses

When my grandmother came from Europe, she brought
all her knowledge of healing "simples" with her, and arnica
was one of her favorites. For the *Arnica montana*, or leopard's
bane of Europe, she found an almost identical American arnica
counterpart. Every so often, she stirred her yellow arnica
flowers into heated lanolin to make a "bruise" ointment.
Sometimes she made an arnica liniment with her own home
vinegar, or created a tincture in some inexpensive brandy or,
more likely, in the case of arnica (since it is applied *externally
only*), out of a better grade of rubbing alcohol.

Medicine Chest Ideas Arnica montana, or the various wild
American arnicas, are just one of the many yellow flowering
plants that I love to use for healing, and most especially for
first aid. The others that come to mind at this point are
marigold (*Calendula officinalis*, or *pot marigold*), chamomile, St.
John's wort, mullein, Solomon's seal, and comfrey.

I keep some form of all of these flowers in my home
medicine chest for first-aid emergencies. Chamomile I use in
flower form for quick infusions, for its antiseptic abilities, and
for its internal quieting abilities. I keep comfrey in root form
for internal or external healing, and I always have a home
comfrey ointment and tincture on hand. One night, recently, I
discovered a sore in my mouth, for instance. I couldn't
imagine how I got one on the inner part of the lower gum, but
I recalled I had been at the dentist that morning for a tooth
cleaning and he had probably scraped the gum. I dabbed

comfrey ointment on the sore. By morning, the abrasion had disappeared.

I keep calendula in a lotion, tincture, ointment, and oil form in the medicine chest. Usually I buy these ready-made from one of the top herbal or homeopathic pharmacies. St. John's wort is a backup for calendula. Mullein flower oil (available from several homeopathic pharmacies) is a must for earaches.

Arnica Needs As for the arnica, I always have some arnica ointment, arnica lotion, arnica tincture, and arnica vinegar on hand for our family. Other medicine chest suggestions are scattered through the book.

Historical Uses The late Father John Kunzle, an herbalist of the last century, considered arnica one of the important healing herbs, and suggested that it be made into an ointment or a tincture in "case of sprains, dislocation and swellings caused by them." Use the undiluted tincture or arnica vinegar as a liniment. Arnica can be diluted in water. Use it as a tea in a foot or arm bath or dip a three-folded cloth into the tincture solution or arnica vinegar, wring it out, and fold the compress over the bruise, pain, or sprain. However, I must warn that *arnica is never to be used on open flesh wounds externally.* Arnica may only be used on *unbroken* skin!

Kunzle, in one of his rare technical suggestions, says to make an "Arnica tincture, use good clean arnica blossoms soaked in alcohol. Place bottle in the sun, or another warm place, for ten days, then strain." (See "Tinctures.")

Ointment Note the directions for making an ointment, or pour about fifteen drops of the tincture into an ounce of anhydrous lanolin, and stir or heat slightly until the tincture is completely distributed and absorbed.

Official Recognition *Arnica montana* was official in various pharmocopoeias in the United States. It was official in the *USP, 1820–51*, and the flowers were official in *USP, 1851–1925*

and in the *NF 1926–1960*. The root was official in the *USP,
1882–1905*. *Remington's Practice of Pharmacy* shows arnica plaster recipes and indicates the tincture was used as an embroca-
tion (liniment) for counterirritant purposes (rubefacient).
When a substance is used as a counterirritant it brings blood to
the surface and breaks up an internal congestion. Mustard
plasters are the most famous and widely used of the counterirritants.

Pain Killer   There is another use for arnica stemming from
another separate branch of medicine: homeopathy. Since this
is a book on folk cures, family remedies, and preventive and
remedial attributes of certain herbs and foods that are herbs, I·
do not wish to embark on a discussion of homeopathy. I
would like to say, though, that although arnica may never be
used internally in its natural form, as a tea, for instance, and
should never be used on open cuts, I have found the
homeopathic pill form of arnica is useful for first-aid shock and
muscular pain. I often use arnica in the 6X size, which is one of
the usual sizes in home homoeopathic kits. I have used it
myself and for family members for shock after accidents. The
British physician Dr. Dorothy Shepard has written two splen-
did books* on her use of various homoeopathic remedies, and
she considers the 6X pill form the "homoeopathic pain killer."

In these books she notes case histories of her successful
use of arnica in its special homoeopathic form (reduced in a
special way so that only a vibration of the plant is left for use).
She claims it to be successful for pain and swelling from
dentistry. Dr. Shepard notes her use of 6X arnica for childbirth, to relieve pain in setting an arm, for concussions,
injuries, falls, blasts, fractures, and dislocations.

While I am describing my own experience with such
homeopathic standbys, and I am quoting Dr. Shepard, I in no
way suggest that you use homoeopathic medicine until you

---

*Shepard, Dorothy, *Magic of the Minimum Dose* and *More Magic of the
Minimum Dose*, Health Science Press, Northhamptonshire, Great Britain.

have studied it further, and conferred with a homoeopathic practitioner-physician.

CAYENNE PEPPER
(Capsicum minimum)

To Bite   Our daughter Caitlin started to call cayenne pepper "red shoes" when she was about three years old, and therein lies a tale that indicates the imaginative versatility of this beloved condiment. But before I tell you that tale, let me give you an idea of the range of health uses for "red-bird" pepper.

Its official name, *Capsicum*, is derived from the Greek word "to bite," and a single use will convince you that the herb is indeed to be treated with delicacy and respect. The surprise, then, is that cayenne, so pungent and biting to the tongue, is nonetheless benign and gentle within the body and is considered by some to be a reliable restorative and internal stimulant.

My personal experience with cayenne goes back to the time when I myself was but three years old and recuperating from a series of children's diseases, topped by a devastating mastoid infection. Having brought me back from death's door by some bold natural cures, Grandma took over the job of building my health back up again.

One of Grandma's edible invigorators was a chutney-like preparation for which I developed quite a fondness at that time. It consisted of thinly sliced, unpeeled cucumbers, crushed shallots and chives, as well as several mashed "bird peppers," all soaked together in lemon juice and then in Madeira wine. I found out years later that this is essentially the recipe for West Indian "Mandram," an Island appetite stimulant and an aid for weak digestion.

Much of the best Capsicum comes from Zanzibar. But a good grade of this red pepper is said to also come from Louisiana. At any rate, this pungent herb was originally brought to Britain in the late 1500s as a condiment from India, where it was also used as one of the many medicinal herbs in Ayurvedic medicine.

Stimulant My own investigations into the historical use of cayenne in Western culture all seem to lead to Vermont-born Samuel Thompson, one of the first ardent proponents of cayenne. Thompson was an interesting lay healer who developed a complete system of herbal and water cures, as well as other natural cures. In a burst of pride (and down-to-earth business sense), he sought to actually patent his herbal cures in the early 1800s, and to everyone's astonishment was given a patent! I don't know how he discovered the stimulating effects of cayenne or if its use as such was already known by local herbalists, but cayenne pepper did come to figure as one of the important herbs in his system.

Despite Thompson's patents, his herbal program leaked out and became a general part of the American *materia medica* of the 1800s. One part of that program usually included, as the second step, a dash of cayenne in a drink to insure internal stimulation.

Swinburne Clymer, in *The Medicines of Nature*, succinctly sums up the distinguished character of our condiment:

> Capsicum increases the power of all other agents, helps the digestion when taken with meals, and arouses all the secreting organs. Whenever a stimulant is indicated, Capsicum may be given with the utmost safety, and should have first consideration. It is indicated in low fevers and prostrating diseases. Capsicum is non-poisonous, and there is no reaction to its use. It is the only natural stimulant worthwhile considering in diarrhea or dysentery with bloody mucus, stools and offensive breath.

Digestive Aid ★ The way to use cayenne as a digestive aid is simply this: Add a tiny pinch (remember that a little goes a long way) to cooked or raw foods, or add a dash to any hot soup or hot tea.

Nutrient Source ★   The herb is a source of vitamin C, and I know that some adventurous souls have learned to add as much as a third of a teaspoon to their daily diet. However, even an infinitesimal amount of cayenne, in food or drink, has an effect on the body, and thus your first experimentations with cayenne dosages should be conservative.

One very effective *energizing* drink is the combination of grape juice with cayenne. I usually add about a quarter of a teaspoon to a quart of unsweetened grape juice, and take this tangy drink on long trips to sustain us on our drive. It is also a delicious, nontoxic drink that can be helpful during school exam periods or at other times when alertness must be maintained for a prolonged period.

Remedies   To combat sore throat, here is a sherry gargle. In this wine I steep everyday kitchen herbs, including cloves, cinnamon, nutmeg, and a little cayenne pepper. It is an aromatic, tasty, and effective antiseptic gargle.

There is also an easy-to-make antiflu cayenne concoction which is a sure winner. Our family has been using it for some time, and it is one of the preparations I demonstrate in the "History and Uses of Herbs for Health" classes I conduct at several colleges. Personally, I like the taste of this cure, but my family does not. Therefore, at the very first school presentation I was surprised to discover that every one of the students in the class not only liked, but loved, the preparation. Perhaps several of them were on the verge of catching a cold that evening, because they seemed to crave the taste. One young woman, Amy, who was indeed coming down with a cold or flu, said that the preparation made her feel better almost immediately. Amy took the leftover preparation home with her that night and later told me that it worked almost miraculously.

Other men and women in my classes have used it to offset the blah feeling that comes on just before a cold or flu, claiming that they feel well the morning after taking the preparation. However, it is strong stuff, and two women with delicate stomachs reported slight stomach cramps on the day after its use. Since this has never happened to me, I don't know if it indicates that they produce more histamine or if the preparation should be buffered with an herbal antispasmodic such as chamomile. But if you have a delicate digestion, take tiny doses and spread them out during the day.

Antiflu Preparation ★

     2   teaspoons cayenne pepper
     1½ teaspoons sea salt, or common salt
     1   cup boiling water
     1   cup apple cider vinegar

Grind together the cayenne pepper and salt to form a paste. Add boiling water (or some strong, strained chamomile tea). Steep and cool. Add the vinegar to the water. Most adults can take between a teaspoon to a tablespoon every half hour. If it seems too strong, dilute it.

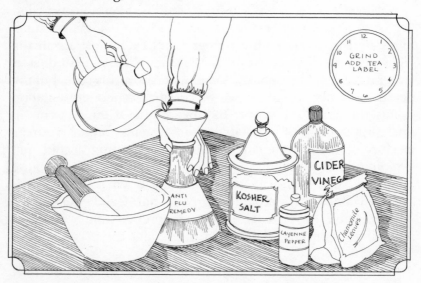

Liniment Another use for cayenne is as a liniment, for it will quickly bring blood to the surface of the skin. Use either apple cider vinegar or alcohol as a base for the liniment, and greatly dilute with rose water, or distilled water. It is also effective to heat the vinegar or the spirits before using them. For a real tingly liniment, I often combine peppermint leaves, a few sprigs of wormwood, rosemary leaves, and a few dashes of cayenne pepper, and steep the preparation in the sun, turning it everyday, for a week or so. Strain off the herbs before using.

Ointment   While cayenne can sometimes smart on the skin, a form of cayenne, oleoresin of capsicum, is often used in professional ointments designed to alleviate rheumatic and other such pains. An early 20th century physician, Dr. W. T. Fernie, reports that such a paste or cayenne ointment "never fails to relieve chronic rheumatism attacks." Since any ointment with cayenne will also stimulate the surface of the hand you use to rub on the ointment, it is wise to use a glove of some kind to apply it.

Persons with sensitive skin, delicate skin, or with known allergic response to stimulating substances should avoid such application.

Bleeding   Cayenne has a sharp effect on the tongue, and will smart on the skin, so it seems like an unlikely candidate as a styptic. For bleeding, I actually prefer calendula (pot marigold) petals either in the form of expressed juice *(Succus calendula)*, or calendula lotion, ointment, or tincture (use a few drops in water for cuts); but a few grains of cayenne will also stop bleeding almost immediately. I once used it on a gushing cut and it arrested the blood flow. American folk use also includes the use of a small amount of cayenne in *hot* water internally to staunch internal bleeding, even from bleeding ulcers; but I have had no personal experience in this regard. I did mention this once while lecturing at a health convention in Madison Square Garden, and asked people to comment on their own experience. One young man said he had drunk the cayenne with cold water, as it was a dire emergency, and that it had worked almost immediately. "It was fantastic," he reported. This use of cayenne for internal bleeding may be useful as a last resort in a crisis on a camping trip, or in some other case where help is remote. But it will be necessary to consult your physician about internal bleeding.

Toothache   A few grains of cayenne will smart on the gum, and in a cavity, but will act as a temporary pain alleviator, until you get to your dentist.

Reaction to Alcohol   Dr. W. T. Fernie reports that diluted tincture of capsicum (cayenne pepper)—a few drops of the tincture plus water in doses of a half teaspoon at a time—will calm agitation from extreme reaction to alcoholic beverages within a few hours, and even promote a calm sleep.

Add sixteen grains of cayenne to every fluid ounce of brandy, gin, or vodka to make your own tincture. This must be steeped for a week or more. Professional tinctures may be purchased from one of several excellent botanical sources. "Nature's Herbs" in Utah has a group of medicinally useful tinctures, including tincture of capsicum (cayenne). (See Resource List.)

Cold Feet ★   Now I want to explain why, when my daughter was a youngster, she called cayenne "red shoes." It's all so simple: during the bitter cold weather, and for ice skating, I sprinkled a combination of cayenne pepper and an inert dusting powder into our shoes. While it may stain the shoes, it protects the feet with a glow of warmth.

Sore Throat   The United States Dispensatory notes one of the most important uses for cayenne is during a malignant sore throat, and in scarlet fever where it is used internally and as a gargle.

Doses   Because of its sharp effect on the tongue, for internal use it is often useful to roll between five to ten grains of the cayenne pepper in some bread or cream cheese to create a pill. For a gargle, add an eighth of a teaspoon of the pepper to a pint of boiling water, or add a few drops of the tincture to rose water. It is a powerful stimulant on the surface of the body, and may be used in small amounts if a mustard plaster is not available, mixed either with apple cider vinegar, or heated whiskey, gin, or vodka, or spirits, to create circulation, in some forms of rheumatism.

Summing Up ★   Cayenne pepper (capsicum) is one of the most important food-herbs, and should be in constant use in your pantry, and always available in your medicine chest. It is a powerful stimulant, producing a sense of heat in the stomach, and a general glow over the body without a narcotic effect. A few grains in hot herbal tea—especially peppermint, chamomile, or linden—will instantly correct sluggish digestion and flatulence. In my experience, cayenne is not only a styptic, but an entirely remarkable body restorative. A few grains added to a herbal tea or water will help reduce many low fevers. A few grains of cayenne in boiling hot water which is then cooled, or added to a combination of common salt and apple cider vinegar, are useful as a gargle, and in tiny doses during the day as a preventative during epidemics of flu or other contagious diseases.

In epidemics and in cases of acute respiratory illness be sure to consult your own physician: cayenne's use as a control for internal or external bleeding is for those health emergencies where no medical or nursing help is immediately available.

In addition to powder form, cayenne (capsicum) may be purchased in tincture or extract form. Use only a few drops in water (up to fifteen drops in a glass of water).

MARIGOLD
(Calendula officinalis)

The pot marigold (Calendula) deserves to be in our everyday medicine chest because it has really remarkable healing powers. I have been using marigold tincture (calendula tincture), lotion and ointment for many years and learned about it from my grandmother, who praised it to the sky as a skin-saving, first-aid herb.

The Romans discovered that marigold bloomed on the first day of each month, and, therefore, named it for the calendar—thus, the Latin term, *Calendula officinalis*. *Officinalis* is the word to indicate official medical abilities as accepted in a pharmacopeia. All the discussion which follows refers to *Calendula officinalis*, and not to any of the hybrid marigolds.

The Skin   Marigold infusion or marigold petal ointment can be used to soothe chapped hands and may be used in infusion form in the baths to reduce body scars, soothe varicose veins, and help control thread veins on the face.

Eczema   Marigold or calendula lotion has been used by many people to help heal painful lesions caused by dry eczema. Here a holistic view is very important; do not tend only to the outer symptoms. Eczema is a problem which often returns when a patient is under stress. To control this health problem, take an intelligent approach to nutrition, utilizing basic vitamin and mineral supplements, add oil to the daily diet—this is important—and drink lots of cleansing herbal teas and lots of pure water. Use cold-water bath therapy.

Mood Elevator   Culpeper and other seventeenth-century herbalists felt that the use of marigold could comfort the spirit. He suggests a chest plaster of marigold steeped in lard, turpentine, and rosin to ease the heart during intense fevers. You can improvise a modern plaster by combining peppermint (menthol and camphor) and marigold ointment as a chest application.

Inflammation   Dip a compress cloth into a strong marigold tea combined with equal parts of apple cider vinegar. Apply it to the inflamed area, and renew it when hot. Wm. Boericke's *Materia Medica with Repertory* has high praise for this delightful garden flower: "Calendula officinalis is a *remarkable healing agent*, applied locally [it is] useful for open wounds, parts that will not heal, ulcers, etc. [It] promotes healthy granulations,

and rapid healing. [It is] haemostatic after tooth extraction . . .
For all *wounds, the greatest healing agent."* (Emphasis mine.)

Vaginal Discharges   Dr. Boericke also mentions that in aque-
ous form, calendula can be used as a douche in leukorrhea.
Leukorrhea refers to various white discharges. The *Merck
Manual* describes leukorrhea as "A nonbloody vaginal discharge which may occur at any age and affects most women at
some time."

Trichomonas vaginitis, a common discharge, has been
known to respond almost immediately to a vinegar douche.
On the other hand, a yeast infection responds to another
natural material—*acidophilus.* Drink acidophilus milk, or take
acidophilus-diluted douches. If you are taking an antibiotic for
an internal discharge or infection, it is very important to *renew*
your internal digestive and vaginal flora with this simple food
substance. It can be obtained at most health-food stores. Some
yogurt strains have been known to have a similar therapeutic
effect on the body. Add diluted calendula tea to either of these
douches.

I often use fresh calendula flowers to reduce the pain and
swelling of a wasp or bee sting, and I use diluted calendula
tincture for broken skin, bleeding, and wounds; calendula
lotion for various kinds of sprains.

Sprains   You can use marigold petals steeped in vinegar for
knee sprains; or you can make a lotion with milk. Simmer a
dozen heads or so of marigolds in 2 cups of milk, steep, strain,
and apply.

Bleeding   I have read that many homeopathic surgeons used
the marigold plant during the Civil War and had much success
with the plant, particularly with the expressed juice of *Succus
calendula* (no pun intended). Incidentally, this particular
"juice" preparation won't keep unless alcohol is added. All
these versions of calendula, particularly tinctures, ointments,
and lotions, can be obtained from such national pharmacies as

Caswell-Massey, Kiehl's, Boericke and Tafel, Luyties, or
Weleda. (See the "Resources" section.)

First Aid   One of the most impressive discussions of the effect
of marigolds in first aid comes from the prolific pen of Dorothy
Shepard, M.D., a British physician. She reports on the use of
calendula by Dr. Petrie Hoyle. She says he used calendula
almost exclusively for "dressing the most filthy wounds" from
the front-line hospital during World War I, and he was
commended by the visiting staff officer for the "clean state of
his patients' wounds, the absence of smell in the wards." He
received much praise for the rapid evacuation and cure of all
kinds of septic wounds among the soldiers. *"All this was due to
the action of the Calendula lotion, and other homeopathic remedies
. . . as no other antiseptics were used in suppurating* [discharging
pus] *wounds."* (Emphasis mine.)

Dr. Shepard was in charge of several different emergency
clinics during her long life as a physician, particularly in poor
neighborhoods. She also worked during the Blitz in London
and used calendula, among other herbs, as one of her
mainstay herbs.

She describes using calendula lotion during a delivery
after labor, both spraying it on the perineum and using wet,
diluted calendula lotion dressings to hasten the healing process. She reported that the midwife was surprised at the fast
healing of the stitches. She also used diluted solution (of the
tincture of calendula) for other wounds wherever the skin was
broken.

> Therefore, in the cases where the skin was broken, I
> used Calendula as a routine measure, and wonder-
> fully quickly it acts. It prevents sepsis [putrefaction].
> Why it does it, I do not know yet; the fact remains it
> does, unless an interfering parent, possessed of a
> little knowledge of first aid, chooses to remove the
> dressing applied at the clinic and uses his own
> favorite antiseptic; then we would find that the
> wound started to fester . . . Let me repeat: No

iodine, no lysol or similar antiseptic, no boracic
fomentations were used any more at the clinic, and
of course no anti-tetanus injections were given, only
plain, usually unboiled water and a few drops of
either Hypericum or Calendula tincture were used. If
the wound or sore was already septic, Hypericum
tincture in the same strength was ordered.

Dr. Shepard used calendula (diluted) even for injuries of
or near the eyes and also used local dressings of calendula for
gunpowder wounds (homeopathic arnica, *internally*, for the
shock) and for all surgical dressings. She also found the herb
effective in dressings after abscesses opened up. Add a few
drops of the tincture of calendula to a cup or more of boiled
water in treating cuts, bruises, and even open wounds. Keep
the dressing wet. Its healing powers are striking.

Older Uses of Marigold

Perspiration   Marigolds were once used to produce perspiration when on the verge of a dangerous illness, particularly
during epidemics of measles and smallpox. Marigold was often
used by English country people either in tea form, or as a
posset. A posset is a drink made with hot milk, and curdled
with either ale or wine. It was sometimes sweetened or spiced.

Henry the VIII   Henry the VIII used marigolds in his personal
recipe, "Medycyne for The Pestilence." In this he used a
handful of marigold, sorrel, burnet, feverfew, and a half-
handful of that old epidemic standby, rue, as well as a few
dragons. (No, not real dragons, but snapdragons.) He wrote,
"This tea, if it is taken before the pimples do apere, then yt will
hele [heal] the syke [sick] person with God's Grace."

For the Heart   Another old use of marigold was to
"strengthen and comfort the hart. . . ." Any number of
seventeenth-century herbals report that marigold flowers were

sold by the barrel to be added to soups, broths, and conserves. Marigold petals can be added to any salad or soup, fresh from the garden.

To Make a Conserve   Conserve is a preserve in which the leaves or flowers are kept intact and whole. Here is a 376-year-old recipe for conserve:

> Take the leaves or flowers of such herbs as you will preserve, make them very cleane, afterward, without anie manner of stamping them, put them whole into some vessell wherein you will keep them, cast upon them a sufficient competence of fine sugar made in pouder; and so set them Sunning in the Vessell. Also in this sort, boyle them at a small fire with Sugar so long as till the Sugar becomes as thick as a Syrup, and after put them in a Vessell.

Toothache and Headache   Stevens says that marigold was once considered a specific remedy for both headache and toothache to country people in England. *The Garden's Labyrinthe* (1577) also describes marigold as a toothache aid: "The juice of Marigold petals mixed with vinegar to be rubbed on gums and teeth becomes a soveraigne remedy for the assuaging of the grevious pain of the teeth."

Red Eyes   Marigold was once considered an excellent remedy for red eyes.

Garden Insect Repellent   All marigolds are excellent aids for "companion planting." They can be planted in many different places in the garden to discourage many insect pests, to repel the asparagus beetle, and to some degree to discourage nematodes and Mexican bean beetles. The nonherb marigolds, dwarf French marigolds *(Tagetes patula)* and African marigolds *(T. erecta)*, especially have a good reputation for discouraging nematodes.

To Dry the Petals   Dry the marigold petals on paper, rather than on screens, as they have a tendency to hold tight to the screen while drying, making it difficult to remove them.

Marigold is available in dried form, as a tincture, pressed juice, ointment, or lotion.

GINGER
[Zingiber officinale]

Ginger grows in the garden or as a window-sill plant and has a spicy, hot characteristic aroma of ginger powder. It is always available in root form in Oriental groceries and fruit stores.

Digestive Aid ★   The fresh ginger, as well as a small amount of the powdered ginger, is stimulating to the digestive organs. While it may seem sharp to the tongue, it seems to quiet and tone the system.

Ginger tea can be used to help with nausea (you'll find that a lot of home spices can be used as an antinausea aid), and the hot tea also helps to relax and calm any internal spasms. In China it is used to overcome mushroom poisoning, and even to check dysentery.

When the body doesn't digest protein well, it often creates too much acid. In extreme cases this is called gastritis, and this uncomfortable problem sometimes occurs after stress or tension. A slice of ginger root or a pinch of ginger powder can be added to tea to calm the body. This can even be helpful in gastritis due to excessive alcohol intake.

Menstrual Aid   Hot ginger tea is useful in stimulating a delayed menstrual period, especially if it is due to a cold. Ginger tea can also help allay severe menstrual cramps.

Detoxifier ★   I have found that ginger tea is a marvelous aid in preventing colds. I frequently use a combination of peppermint, a pinch of ginger, and a pinch of clove powder, or two bruised cloves. Chamomile tea with grated ginger, honey, and lemon is particularly soothing for laryngitis or bronchitis. Ginger is one of the useful herbs during the winter, as it will help to keep the body warm and stimulated. You can certainly add it to any herbal drink during flu weather. However, remember that for flu prevention there is nothing like cayenne pepper or cinnamon bark or cinnamon oil tea.

Antipain—Circulation Aid   Our family has been using grated ginger baths for years. A small amount (and remember, ginger, like cayenne, quickly brings the blood to the surface, and thus must be used in moderation, until the body learns to tolerate it) goes a long way. Ginger baths are great for circulation, and will decrease muscle soreness and muscle stiffness.

To create a tea, use a pinch to a tablespoon of the powder, or grate or slice the fresh root and simmer until there is a yellowish water. Add this tea to the bath. This bath is wonderfully warming and is just the item to use when you want to cut down on your fuel bills. Just jump right into bed after taking the bath, and you'll stay warm for hours afterward.

For pain, you can also soak cloths in ginger tea and apply them directly to the area of pain.

Ginger Ale   I make a home ginger ale—and it is delicious and stimulating as well as nutritious. Wash and chop a medium-sized ginger root. Add a quart of water and simmer until the water is a strong, dark-yellow color. Cool. Strain out the ginger, add honey to taste, and place in a large clean bottle. Add carbonated Perrier or similar type water. Cap or cork.

Ginger Soda   Use the above recipe, but add any unsweetened fruit juice—or, if you would like to try a slightly more difficult home project, one that provides its own carbonation, use this combination (you will have to have a large container, cheesecloth, and be able to eventually cork the bottles):

4   gallons boiling water
½   cup cold water
2   tablespoons yeast
6   lemons
4   cups honey
3   ounces or 6 tablespoons bruised ginger
    root
    bottles and corks

Boil the water. Reserve and cool.

Add the yeast to ½ cup of water. Reserve. Wash—in fact, scrub—the lemons. Take out the pits, and cut up with rind into little pieces.

Combine the honey and the ginger root, lemons and yeast. Add the water.

I use an old stone crock for this, as it has a spigot. Cover the stock with cheesecloth so that your soda can bubble up. Wait twenty-four hours. Strain, bottle, and lightly cork. You can use old sterilized soda or wine bottles. Put the soda into an old refrigerator or in a cool cellar, as otherwise it becomes "ale."

Ginger and Honey Candy   My grandmother made this candy; this recipe makes about two pounds:

1   pound honey—the darker the better
1   pound walnuts—shelled and chopped
    coarsely
½   teaspoon ginger

Simmer the honey over low heat and add the walnuts and the ginger. Stir for forty-five minutes over very low heat.

Butter a large platter and pour the candy. Take it away from the heat, and let it stand for a few hours. This can be cut into different shapes with a wet knife.

Candied Ginger   Cut up a large, clean ginger root into bite-sized slices, and simmer them in a half pound of honey. Do not add water.

GINSENG
(Panax schinseng)

"What is ginseng?" This is one of the most frequent questions I am asked these days, and although I always feel slightly astonished that the questioner has never heard of ginseng before, I recall my own amazement of about fifteen years ago.

I was standing at the counter of Kiehl's, one of New York's old-fashioned herb emporiums, when I heard a very distinguished-looking man next to me order $100 worth of ginseng. That was a lot of ginseng and a lot of money, so I turned to watch him, and I finally dared to ask, "What do you do with all that ginseng?"

He explained, "I'm a professor at a midwestern university, and I do a lot of public speaking around the country. My wife is a well-known pianist. Right before each lecture engagement I take a capsule of the ginseng in hot water. My wife takes two capsules before each concert. We find that the ginseng sharpens our memory and enhances our delivery. We also use it whenever we are feeling run down. And it's great for getting rid of coughs!"

I whistled with astonishment. Was ginseng *(Panax schinseng)* really a panacea as its name implied? On his say-so and on the assurance from the reputable Kiehl men that ginseng wasn't at all addictive, I purchased an ounce. We've had ginseng in the house ever since.

Our experience with ginseng is that it is a terrific tonic and pick-me-up. It does indeed sharpen the memory for very special occasions, is a specific for coughs, and a help (along with vitamin C and other herbs) in warding off a cold. ★

It appears to be a mild stimulant for the central nervous system, and although in the Far East it seems to be used for children, too, when they need it, like all stimulants it should always be used in great moderation.

There is no doubt that the Chinese, the Koreans, and the

Japanese, indeed most of the peoples of the Far East, consider this white man-shaped root a medicinal panacea. They use it for all kinds of respiratory and inflammatory conditions and for many blood diseases. It is considered an effective normalizing medicine and a great help to someone who is very ill. For that reason, even a poor Asian will sell a family treasure to buy some ginseng for a beloved one who is extremely sick. The ginseng is then cooked with chicken, and the soup used again and again as a restorative broth. It is one of the two herbs most frequently used in the traditional herbal medicine of the Far East.

The wealthy and ambitious, however, often use ginseng every day. Some chew roots; some use the powder in hot tea; others use the extract. In Korea and Japan the "red" ginseng is considered the most valuable and the most effective. In all cases, Korean, Japanese, and Chinese men seem to think that in using ginseng they will preserve and enhance their sexual prowess. My theory is that the root works as a body toner. And when you feel good, everything looks rosy—everything you do is effective.

One of the greatest travel adventures of my life occurred recently when I received an invitation to attend the First International Ginseng Conference in Seoul. Very formal papers by top scientists from America, Germany, the Bahamas, Sweden, Korea, and Japan were presented. The other two invited American guests had become ill at the last minute, so I was the only American writer there.

The entire conference, held at the elegant and continental Chosun Hotel in Seoul, was conducted in English, with simultaneous translations into Japanese, Chinese, Korean, and, I suppose, several other languages of the Orient, since most of the delegates were from the Far East.

Cultivation   Ginseng, I discovered, takes six years to mature and must be carefully cultivated under precise forest conditions. The composition of the soil (and during the conference I heard many, many reports on this *yakto*, or soil, for medicinal plants), the planting of the mysterious and unique seeds, and a year later, the transplanting of the strongest seedlings are crucial. The nurturing and protection given to the plants (the plants are consistently shielded from the sun by angled awnings of straw), the ritual of the harvest, the excitement of selecting the roots, the routine of the precise sorting were carefully explained and then brilliantly depicted in a fine film (in English) and in field trips.

Experiments   There were two interesting reports from the Faculty of Pharmaceutical Sciences, University of Tokyo, one by Dr. Professor S. Shibata, another by Dr. Professor K. Takagi.

Later, in Tokyo, at the pharmacy labs where the experiments took place, I interviewed Professor Takagi as well as Dr. H. Saito, his assistant. They showed me how they worked and how the laboratory mice were aided in recovery and retention of information when given ginseng fraction (Ginsenocide, a chemical part of the root). "There was significant antifatigue reaction with the mice," Dr. Professor Takagi summed up. He also said that Korean ginseng was more of a stimulant than Japanese ginseng. "Also we learned in our experiments that ginseng aids in the acceleration and acquisition of learning."

Another important report presented, one which was enthusiastically received by all the journalists, was from Dr. Finn Sandberg, Faculty of Pharmacy and Faculty of Medicine, Uppsala University, Sweden. In the Sandberg double-blind test, conducted with healthy Swedish college students over a period of thirty-three consecutive days, two ginseng preparations were tested together with a placebo (an inert pill which looks like the test pill). Two tests were given to three groups of student volunteers, ten to a group, five male, five female. These were divided into random groups and were given one capsule morning and evening of either of the ginseng preparations and/or placebo.

The tests consisted of a spiral maze test and a letter crossover test. The spiral maze method, developed in Britain, requires moving a pen along a spiral without touching fifty-four small rings in the maze. The elbows of the students had to be elevated at all times.

The letter constellation test consisted of a five-minute test in which each student had to cross each letter that was situated between two columns, cross each similar letter, and cross each pair of letters.

Sandberg, an international expert on medicinal plants who has worked for UNESCO in Pakistan, Africa, and the Far East, noted that the "statistical treatment of the data obtained showed a significant effect of both preparations."

During a luncheon interview, Professor Sandberg told me that it was difficult for his test to show definitive results because the action of the ginseng is actually mild. He felt, however, that there was no doubt that the students who took the two ginseng preparations worked faster and achieved better results.

Sandberg also told me he considered ginseng a stimulant. He uses it on all his travels and whenever needed in his daily life. "When I am in any particular stress, I take pills of ginseng for three or four weeks. Then I stop. I take it at intervals whenever I feel the need." ★

Other papers of interest were those of the Swiss K. H. Rueckert, who found that the swimming performance of ginseng-treated mice surpassed that of untreated mice, and the observations of I. M. Popov, M.D., of the Bahamas on the ginseng reaction of various patients at the Renaissance Revitalization Center. "A constant increase of favorable effects of different therapies have been found in the majority of treated cases without ever encountering undesirable side effects"— meaning he likes ginseng for most of his patients and uses it all the time and finds no side reactions.

Field Trip   One of the most exciting highlights to the Korean trip was the visit to the ginseng growing fields. We rolled by bus through the city and into the country, passing village after village. On the way to the fields that were to be dug up for us that day, we noted many small ginseng farms. Ginseng can be grown only under supervised forest conditions; thatched straw awnings are the mark of these farms.

The production of raw ginseng is expected to be increased to 15,700,000 kilograms by 1981. In prior centuries, Korean ginseng was exported mainly to China. Today it also goes to Europe, Africa, the Middle East, North and South America. A million dollars of ginseng in various forms of powder, extract, and tea comes from Korea into the United States each year.

After an hour's ride, the buses finally stopped on the edge of a ginseng farm. The fields had been stripped of the thatched awnings, and now we were able to see several sorting areas with many farming women and children sitting under a canopy and, in the fields, a tall bamboo guardhouse where peasants guarded the crop. White-clad, white-capped farmers now extracted the ginseng with a special claw-like instrument, as tenderly (and tensely) as porcupines make love. Other white-clad farmers with square black hats placed the roots in huge baskets and carried the baskets to the sorting canopy. Here the women, each in elaborate, colorful head scarfs, carefully placed the fresh roots into color, shape, and size groups. The best are then sold to the government for their red ginseng.

Afterwards I talked for a while with Johan Lamoral, a Belgian journalist with *Gazet van Antwerpen*, who said, "Although ginseng is thousands of years old, many people around the world, including Europeans, discovered the tonic herb only recently, and still wonder about the medical effectiveness of the item. As for the Belgians, they heard about ginseng from the Belgian soldiers returning from the Korean War. The story about the substance awoke many Belgians and people in other European countries to the mysterious effects of ginseng. Although scientific research is still to be made on the medical herb, and European scientists are still skeptical of its effectiveness, no one seems to doubt its revitalizing power."

Body Regulator ★ Early in Chinese herb pharmacy, ginseng was used as a body regulator. One modern physician, Park Seung-Ku, M.D., trained in both Western and "traditional" medicine, explained to me, "The function of herb drugs is principally to coordinate various functions of the human body. Health exists when K1 (energy) and Hyol (blood), or yin (negative) and yang (positive), maintain their proper balance. Disease occurs when there is a loss of balance. In treating disease with herb drugs, the theory is to bring the energy and blood level into balance again." A little bit goes a long way, I have found.

Energy and Ginseng ★ There are many ways to achieve energy when you are fatigued: external baths, certain self- and formal-massage points, pressure points, vitamins, minerals, and mental relaxation methods. Among the many natural substances that can be used to advantage is ginseng. Take a pinch of the powder in a cup of hot water and drink it. Or use one of the prepared tea extracts, or less than an eighth of a teaspoon of the extract, or a capsule of the powdered root, or chew a piece of the raw root.

You do not need large doses of ginseng to help you restore flagging energy. Less is more: tiny doses are best.

Ginseng is presently available in dried root form, tincture, powder, and extract.

ROSEMARY
(Rosmarinus officinalis)

Whenever I write of any herb I seem to say, "This one is my favorite." But in some ways it is true. Herbs are a little like children: They take on personalities, and you love each one for their individual qualities.

Take rosemary, for instance. Today it is considered a culinary aid, but it was once regarded as one of the great cure-all herbs. It was mentioned for its medical and cosmetic powers by Pliny, by Dioscordes, by Galen, and revered by the early Arab physicians. We know today that it is an antiseptic, a gentle stimulant to the entire body, a wonderfully aromatic garden aid, a headache dispeller, a folk-medicine heart tonic, and, and, and . . . the list for this ancient cure-all goes on. But before I share all the virtues of the medical rosemary, let me share a special visual and olfactory one.

Have you ever traveled along the Mediterranean shores? I hope that you can sometime in your future, for one of my most pleasant memories of Italian shores is the pervasive, heady aroma of the evergreen, blue-flowered, wild rosemary. Rosemary loves rocky mountainsides and cliffs, and because it grows so well and so near the sea, *Rosmarinus* means "dew of the sea," or "sea spray."

Breath Aid ★ John Gerard, in his ancient herbal, mentions that rosemary is useful in keeping the breath sweet and clean. He advises drinking the distilled water of the flowers early in the morning and last thing at night. Culpeper suggests eating the flowers every morning, while fasting, with bread and salt: "It helps dim eyes, and procures a clear sight."

I make an inexpensive rosemary-spice-sherry gargle that you might like to try. If you haven't a sprig of fresh rosemary, use a pinch of the dried herb. I purchase a cheap sherry, and add a pinch each of cloves, cinnamon, anise seed, and a dust or two of mace, plus the rosemary. I steep, turn and shake the herbs in the sherry for a week or so, then strain them out. It's cheaper than most mouthwashes, and twice as effective and delicious. It is a great gift, by the way. Don't forget to label it, although I must confess that these items added to any wine only enhance its taste and act in a stimulating way on the body. (See Section Three.)

Memory Some herbs, such as elder or rosemary, seem to evoke mystery and symbolism among our ancient forebears. Do you recall the phrase, "Rosemary, that's for remembrance?" Well, rosemary was thought to sharpen the memory. It was also thought to relate to fidelity. Thus, a sprig of aromatic rosemary was always woven into a bride's headdress.

Disease Prevention ★ Rosemary was also thought to be one of the several herbs that could help ward off disease, and it is contained in many a family recipe and involved with many legendary recipes during the bubonic plague. Sprigs of fresh rosemary and fresh rue were always placed next to the judges in the dock and strewn about the English courts. It was believed they prevented diseases from spreading. No wonder a 1550 herbal says to drink a tea of rosemary flowers, "for it is much worth against all evyls in the body."

Because there was a strong belief in rosemary's antidisease abilities, each mourner was handed a sprig of fresh rosemary at a funeral, to have, to hold, and then drop on the coffin. "Dry up your tears, and stick rosemary on this fair corse [sic]," Father Lawrence says in *Romeo and Juliet*.

Restorative ★   But to our ancestors, rosemary had still other uses. My own grandmother had a strong feeling about the restorative abilities of this herb; she often suggested it for morning tea, and, as do the English herbalists (apparently this feeling pervaded all of Europe), she believed that rosemary could "comfort the brain."

Certainly, grandmother believed in rosemary for headaches, and, along with chamomile and linden, she liked rosemary for all sorts of sudden nervous upsets.

Because my grandmother had been rescued by the gypsies when she was young, she believed some of their superstitions. One was that a sprig of rosemary under a pillow could prevent children's nightmares.

Grandmother said that rosemary could prevent a miscarriage. However, many of the English herbalists indicate a contrary use of the herb—to bring on a delayed period! That's one of the interesting things about herbs—the contradictory uses. But then, I often wonder, how did the millions who lived before us actually discover the many uses of each herb?

Rosemary leaves can be used as a tonic tea, to stimulate and strengthen the system after an illness or when one is exhausted. Rosemary leaves added to wine are said to strengthen the heart and prevent the swelling of the ankles so common with certain heart conditions. Also, rosemary can act as a diuretic by releaseing fluid from the system. Kunzle used rosemary to stimulate menstruation, for headaches, nerves, strengthening after exhaustion, nervous heart troubles, stomach diseases, a diuretic, and even congestion of the liver.

Grandmother had several ways to prepare rosemary-steeped wine. For her heart cordial, she used a white wine.

I have had very positive reactions to her old tonic wine. We make it in my "History and Uses of Herbs for Health" classes. Since it will hold well, I use a full-bodied, red wine, a Madeira. Many students use the wine when they feel ill. One student had an undetermined flu-like illness. She said this tonic wine was the only food she could tolerate. "It saved me during those two home-bound weeks."

Cold, Headaches, Stomach Spasms   Add a small amount of fresh, or a pinch of dried, rosemary to other herbal teas. It combines well with sage, with lavender (also good against headaches), and, of course, it can be combined with the old standbys for stomach spasms—chamomile or peppermint.

External Stimulant ★   Rosemary is especially stimulating for the skin, and, therefore, is a wonderful scalp aid, too. It can be added to shampoos and rinses to prevent dandruff and to strengthen the hair and make it glisten. It is particularly good for those with dark hair.

I have mentioned the tonic effect of rosemary on the skin, and aside from the excellent counterirritants like mustard, wintergreen, and the like, rosemary should take its place as a wonderful yet rather gentle external stimulant. For this reason, it can be added in strong tea form to the bath water to help with sluggish circulation, and it can be added to a steam facial to activate a sluggish, sallow complexion.

One link with the medieval past that I like is the Queen of Hungary water. The Hungarian Queen Elizabeth is said to have been cured of paralysis by the continued use of rosemary on her limbs, and the Imperial Library in Vienna is said to have a formula for Queen of Hungary water written in the Queen's own hand in 1235. This water was sold all over Europe, was found in many European apothecaries, and was also sold by certain groups of European gypsies as a face beautifier and cure-all.

This famous water was distilled from the flowers of rosemary. But you can get some of the same external effect, some old pharmacy books say, from the leaves, since the camphorous oil of rosemary is in the leaves. The original water was made with a pound or more of the flowers in a gallon of white wine, then distilled again. You could try your own version with homegrown rosemary leaves steeped in a white wine. It makes a stimulating rub. Some allergic people may be sensitive to rosemary oil on the skin, however, so experiment cautiously.

Rosemary can be obtained in oil, tincture, dried form, or in pressed herbal juice.

THE THREE C'S: CLOVES, CINNAMON, CARAWAY

Cloves *[Eugenica caryophyllata]*

Pomander—An Aromatic Insect Repellent Hoist those unwanted moths on a clove petard by studding a thin-skinned orange with the aromatic flower buds from the evergreen clove tree. The best, the darkest, the strongest, and the most aromatic of these brown studs are said to come from the Moluccas or Spice Islands.

Fragrant balls of aromatics were once used as an antidote to disease. Pomanders were often made with apples, but oranges were considered even more helpful against pestilence. Today these spicy balls, made either with oranges, apples, lemons, limes, or kumquats, are mainly used as insect repellents in closets or clothes drawers.

Studding the Pomander Pierce a few holes in the orange with a thin steel nail or large darning needle and insert a group of cloves at a time until the orange is completely covered in concentric circles of cloves. Depending on the size of the fruit and the size of the cloves (the largest are best), this may take several hours (a great rainy-day group activity). Use a thimble to push large cloves into the rind.

Next sprinkle the clove-studded fruit with your favorite spice blend. An easy home mixture is a combination of these blended powders: four tablespoons of cloves, six tablespoons of nutmeg, one-half tablespoon of ginger, and one tablespoon of orris root (needed as a fixative). Be careful to cover the area between the cloves, so that the juices of the fruit and the spices will mingle and become one.

Turn the clove-orange from time to time until the fruit dries and shrivels. Encase it in a cheesecloth or open mesh nylon cloth, and hang in a closet to dry. After several weeks, tie the orange with a narrow red velvet ribbon, crossing at the base. Place a large looped bow on the top, and hang the orange in a clothes closet or use it in a drawer with woolen sweaters.

These spice-impregnated fruits are anathema to insects. They last for a lifetime and can be revitalized by redipping into the same aromatic concoction.

Clove Gargle　We have a custom of making a rich hot wine grog on New Year's Day. These same spices, without the sweetener and in sherry, can be transformed into a good-tasting, strong antiseptic gargle for sore throat or for mouth rinsing.

You can use your leftover wine for a mouthwash if you like. The light wines are best; the others have too much body.

> 1　pint (inexpensive) sherry
> 1　ounce (2 tablespoons) bruised cloves
> ½　ounce (1 tablespoon) bruised cinnamon
> 　　pinch of bruised caraway seeds
> 　　lavender water—optional, to be used later

Steep the spices and seeds in the sherry. Keep the mixture in a dark closet. Shake it as often as you can. After a week or two strain out the herbs (I have left them in and it doesn't do any harm, but eventually they get mushy and stringy). Add a few drops of lavender water or lotion to the gargle for aroma. To use the gargle for sore throat, add about a teaspoon to a tablespoon of the wine to a glass of water.

Clove Oil Anesthetic   When you scrape or bruise cloves, you release a valuable, volatile oil which can be a temporary skin anesthetic. That is why whole bruised cloves can be rolled in the mouth (or first soaked in hot honey) for temporary toothache aid. Clove oil can be purchased in drugstores but be careful how you use it—it is extremely strong on the skin. However, a tiny bit can be added to liquid and pure anhydrous lanolin to relieve topical irritability of eczema. Some allergic people may be sensitive to clove oil so be *very* cautious in using it.

Clove oil plus zinc oxide (ointment) is still sometimes used by dentists for temporary fillings, and to disinfect depulped root canals before permanent restoration of a tooth.

To make your own clove oil, shove a handful of the largest and the darkest bruised cloves into olive oil until the jar is full. Strain out the cloves after a week, save the oil, and repeat the process until the oil is saturated with newly released clove oil.

Sleep Aid   This volatile oil from cloves can also be released by bruising and steeping the cloves in boiling water, and then simmering them for a few minutes. When simmering, do not allow the water to be reduced too much, as this creates a stronger extract of cloves. one which may be too strong in its sleep effect. However, a teaspoon to a cup of boiling water will produce a mild and slightly sedative tea. You can also add other sleep-rewarding herbs such as chamomile, linden, or sage. This tea can also be used as a temporary toothache aid.

Depression   Clove tea or bruised cloves added to such herbal teas as chamomile, linden, or peppermint can often help lift people out of mild depressions. Thus, it is a good idea to use a clove or two in the tea of those who tend to be depressed.

Nausea Aid   Cloves act less upon the system at large than on the part to which they are immediately applied. They are, therefore, very useful in digestive problems—weak digestion or nausea—and a clove tea or bruised cloves added to other herbal teas will relieve nausea and vomiting, correct flatulence, and excite "languid" digestion. They are also very valuable in other medicinal preparations to assist the action of other herbs. Cloves may be tried for digestive problems along with cinnamon, nutmeg, cardamom, caraway, fennel, and anise.

Finger Cut An ordinary cut, particularly a paper cut on a finger, can be extremely painful. Here's my father's favorite remedy: Wet your finger, and dip it into powdered cloves. The pain will quickly disappear. This is because cloves have a special ability to slightly anesthetize the skin.

Cinnamon

The inner bark of the shoots of the cinnamon tree is a powerful local stimulant which acts to ease the stomach and relieve spasms; it is also a mild astringent. Like cloves it acts in a local rather than in a general way on the body. Cinnamon is used a good deal in herbal medicine to overcome the unpleasant odors of certain herbs and to act as a partner with other herbs. It is helpful in diarrhea and is said to be helpful for children in bedwetting and as sleep medicine for children. Cinnamon, with other herbs, is an antinausea aid. It is an old English flu-preventive.

Flu-Preventive ★ Add five drops of true cinnamon oil to a tablespoon of water, and use it several times a day at the very onset of a flu epidemic or immediately after you think you have been exposed to flu. This remedy was used with great effectiveness by English physicians at the turn of this century. It is important to use this remedy before the flu sets in; otherwise, it seems to have no effect.

To create a less effective home version of this oil, bruise the cinnamon bark and "release" in simmering boiled water, or in brandy.

Some allergic people may be sensitive to cinnamon oil.

Pregnancy Aid   Use a small amount of the bruised bark in any mild herbal tea (chamomile or linden would be fine) one hour before bedtime.

> 1   ounce (2 tablespoons) cinnamon bark (or powder)
> 1½ pints distilled water

Boil the water and steep the cinnamon bark in it for fifteen minutes or more. Take one teaspoon at a time one hour before meals for nausea or vomiting, or to relieve flatulence. Use small amounts at first to check for possible sensitivity during pregnancy.

Cinnamon Taste   I always keep a jar of dried cinnamon bark on my kitchen pantry shelf. When I want to add the tingly, cleansing taste of cinnamon to other herbal teas, I merely bruise a small piece of the bark on a grater or with my mortar and pestle. This helps to release some of the tantalizing cinnamon oil. This bark need not be thrown away immediately, as it can be used and reused several times, up to about five times.

Antinausea   The use of cinnamon goes back in all ancient history. It is said that King Solomon recommended its use and it may have been brought by Arabs to the Phoenicians, Greeks, and Romans. It is still freely used in the Near East. For families plagued by weak digestion or nausea problems, here is the compound powder of cinnamon. Keep it in a labeled jar, ready for use.

> 3   small thin sticks, or 1 stick (about 6″) cinnamon bark
> 1   tablespoon (about 8 seeds) cardamom seed
> 1   tablespoon (1 medium nutmeg) nutmeg

Grind the bark and the seeds together in a nut grinder,

coffee grinder, or blender. Place the mixture in a jar. Label:
Antinausea. Use ¼ teaspoon to one cup hot tea for an adult,
and a tiny pinch of the powder to one cup hot tea (then cool)
for a child.

Cramps Make up a hot tea, bruise some cinnamon bark, or
add powdered cinnamon (though the powder in a hot drink
tends to look like slush). Add honey.

Caraway
[Carum carvi]

Digestion This tasty fruit which we all call a seed is found in
rye bread partly because it is helpful in digestion. Add a few
drops of caraway oil to a teaspoon of hot water for flatulence
and indigestion. Or use the after-dinner liquor, Kümmel,
made from caraway seed. It has a marvelous aroma and taste.
      Anise and caraway oil (if the oils are not available, the two
combined bruised seeds can be steeped in boiling water) are
known to have helped stomach spasms. Together they act as
an antiseptic and stimulant.
      To help with digestive problems in infants, make either a
caraway milk or caraway julep.

Caraway Milk For colic, crush some seeds and simmer them
in milk for about twenty minutes. Strain, and give the liquid to
the child. This can also be used for adult colic.

Caraway Julep Steep two tablespoons of the bruised seeds
for six hours in a pint of cold water. Strain the liquid, and give
it to the infant in tiny, child-sized teaspoons to alleviate colic or
digestive problems. (See also "Favorite Herb Tea Blends.")

Poultices When I was a child I remember my father making
caraway and hot bread poultices for earaches. Bruised and
simmered caraway tea may also be used to relieve swellings of
the breasts or testicles. These health problems should be
investigated by a physician to avoid future complications.

DANDELION, CHICORY, AND CHICKWEED

Dandelion
[Taraxacum officinale]

Lincoln used to say that God must have loved the little people, he made so many of them, and he certainly must have loved the thousands of wildflowers and useful weeds that grow unheralded, uncared for, even despised. One of my very favorite wildflowers is the dandelion. Perhaps if it were as rare as the showy orchid, we would pay more attention to it, but because it grows everywhere, including the middle of our lawns, we ignore it as a pest.

Food   Oddly enough this seeming pest is a favorite eating herb of many cultures, and I have passed down many highways in the spring and noted whole families collecting the young dandelion leaves. In April the leaves can be picked as they push through the earth, and after rinsing they can be mixed with toasted soy bits, lemon, oil, a touch of nutmeg, and several hardboiled eggs to make a delicious and healthful spring lunch.

Neutralizer ★   The salts in dandelion act to neutralize the acids in the blood, and thus dandelion is considered a cleansing tonic. But the leaves have to be gathered when they are young, otherwise they are too bitter. Later in the season you can infuse the tops (flowers and some leaves) into an old-fashioned curative tea, useful for biliousness and for reducing swelling in the ankles. Use a handful of the tops to a pint of boiling water. Steep for ten minutes or so, strain, and add honey. Drink this several times a day.

Liver   The bitter dandelion *root* is beloved in folk medicine and it is especially used to stimulate a sluggish liver. The old recipes say to drink from two to four ounces. Simmer two ounces of the freshly sliced root in two pints of water until the water is reduced to one pint. Add one ounce of compound tincture of horseradish (herbal pharmacies have it).

Coffee   Coffee made from dandelion root is available in some health-food stores. It is thought to be a liver cleanser and also has a tonic effect on the pancreas, the spleen, and the female organs.

To make your own dandelion root coffee, gather some fresh root. Wash it, and allow it to dry in a warm place. When it is shriveled, roast it slightly and grind it into a fine powder by using your food processor, a nut grinder, or an old-fashioned hand grinder. To make the coffee, add a cup of boiling water to each teaspoon of the powder. This is a bitter drink, but one with no side effects and no acid.

Gallstones   Dandelion is also an old folk remedy for gall-stones. To help with this problem, the following combination was recommended by ancient herbalists: one ounce each of dandelion root, parsley root, lemon balm, with a half ounce each of licorice root and ginger root. Add two quarts of boiling water, simmer down to one quart, strain the liquid, and drink a half glass every two hours. Be sure to check this problem with a physician.

China   "The "barefoot doctors" of China use the whole dandelion plant in their healing practices. The leaves and the tops are simmered together in a decoction, or they are crushed as a poultice on breast abscesses (this poultice can be used on boils or abscesses on other parts of the body, or added to honeysuckle flowers).

Chicory
[Cichorium intybus]

Chicory is another fine if lowly weed, with pale, lovely blue flowers. This daisy-petaled flower blossoms from July to

September, emerging each morning and fading by noon all along waysides and meadows.

Food   As with dandelion, the young tender leaves are used in summer salads or blanched as a vegetable. But—again as with dandelion—use the plant before the flowers form, otherwise it will taste too bitter.

Coffee   The root has been used for centuries as "coffee" or a coffee extender in the same way as described for dandelion root. I first came across chicory coffee in the French Quarter in New Orleans. It is quite bitter but, like the dandelion, is also a mild tonic, a liver cleanser, and is slightly laxative and mildly diuretic (releases retained fluids).

As you undoubtedly know by now, true coffee is not only expensive, but should be used only in moderation. There seems to be a connection between high coffee intake and heart attacks. You should not drink coffee if you have high blood pressure, and it is a virtual poison for arthritis and other systemic disease sufferers. (Oddly enough, coffee enemas help to depoison and detoxify the body. Don't use them too often; the action is immediate and strong.)

Use all sorts of herbal teas as coffee replacement. Learn to combine the various mints along with cloves, a dash of cinnamon, and nutmeg. Use honey and vanilla extract (there are some wonderful pure ones on the market) with these teas, or with linden, which makes another fine herbal drink. Chamomile will relax you and overcome spasms.

Essence   Besides using the leaves of chicory for salads or a cooked green, and the root for a hot beverage, there is still another unique and charming use for chicory—this time for the flowers. Pick them early in the day, and let them soak in fresh water in the sun. Strain the liquid. Store the essence of the water, and add a few drops of it to the tea of those who are on a crying jag, or unduly possessive and overcritical of others! Chicory is an integral part of the (Dr. Edward) *Bach Flower Remedies*.

Chickweed
[Stellaria media]

Once we've talked about chicory, can chickweed be far behind? I say this with a touch of amusement, as most people just can't seem to separate these two similar-sounding weeds. It reminds me of that delightful Hoffenstein poem: "Some people can/Some people can't/Tell the difference between/Gary Cooper and Cary Grant."

Chickweed has half-inch whitish flowers and is like a creeper. It is called chickweed because the chickens and birds love it so much!

Food This lowly plant—found along waysides and on so many lawns—is an excellent herb of many uses. A Swiss herbalist says that fresh chickweed can be prepared like spinach, is a wonderful heart strengthener, and also brings back vigor and strength to those who are recovering from an illness. As children, we were sometimes given drinks of chickweed to cleanse the system and overcome a fever.

Inflammation Chickweed can be crushed and applied to wounds and has the virtue of taking away the heat in any inflammation. There is one other important use chickweed has in addition to the benefits just named: its efficacy as a poultice. The fresh leaves can be applied to the skin for any sort of swelling or skin problem. In the case of intense heat caused by an inflammation, crush the leaves, attach them to the heated area, and place a large cabbage leaf or romaine lettuce leaf over this poultice. The chickweed will soon absorb the heat of any inflammation. Keep on replacing the poultice with fresh chickweed.

Ointment I like to make up a chickweed ointment, just as my grandmother did, by melting the leaves in a quarter pound or so of anhydrous lanolin. I bake it in the oven for several hours, then skim off the burnt herb. My grandmother used this ointment on sore legs and for rheumatic pains.

HONEY: AMBROSIA MEDICINE

That delicious and versatile orange fluid, "that ambrosia of the gods" we call honey, was mankind's first sweet. Our friends the honey bees extract nectar from flowers—and, incidentally, the color, the taste, and the aroma of the honey are derived from the type of flower they feed on. In a mysterious process only recently understood, the bees carry the nectar in a honey sac, wherein special enzymes break down the complex sucrose sugar into two simple sugars: fructose and glucose. This fluid is deposited in open cells in the beehive. The next step, nature's first air conditioning surely, is the evaporation of the excess water brought about by the continuous moving wings of working bees. When the right sugary consistency is reached, each cell is capped with wax. Since each group of bees needs only 400–500 pounds of the honey for themselves, the rest can be collected and used. But still it takes about a thousand trips back from the flower to hive, and sometimes thousands of miles, to produce only two tablespoons of honey!

Each country—and each area within a country—tends to have a distinctive type of honey. While it is easier to cook with the light honeys, it is said that the dark honeys are somewhat more effective for health. While the bees in America tend to produce very light clover honey, there are also many other, darker honeys. Much of the linden honey comes from Czechoslovakia, lavender honey from France, and wild rose honey from Greece. If you have hayfever, you might try eating honeycomb of the plant substance you are allergic to or the honey produced nearest to your home. (Honeys are labeled as to flower and origin.) Because honey is produced from flowers, it can sometimes act as an antihistamine.

Honey for Food-Ceremony-Medicine   We know, of course,

that primitive man used honey as a food. There is in fact a drawing, believed to be 20,000 years old, on the walls of a cave in Spain, that shows a man reaching for a beehive high on a stone cliff. Anthropologists also know that honey is still used in many religious ceremonies among primitive people in New Guinea, Africa, South America, and New Zealand. We do not know much about the use of honey as medicine, except by ancient Hebrews and Egyptians, but honey may have been used as a salve in every one of the many cultures that utilized it as a food. Certainly we must consider also the antifatigue ability of honey as possible medicine and its use in many cultures where people are long-lived. Do not use uncooked, unpasteurized honey for newborn infants, as it may create a fatal diarrhea. Otherwise, this type of honey is preferred.

Healing Power of Honey   We always used honey on minor sores when I was a child, and I still find that a tiny eruption around or in the mouth can be quickly healed with honey. I tend to combine comfrey with honey for this, but honey alone acts both to heal and to destroy bacteria with or without another plant or greasy substance.

In addition to various mentions of the healing power of honey in the Bible, the most interesting medical notes on ancient medicine come from the records of the Egyptians who were—medically speaking—honey addicts. Indeed no fewer than 500 out of 900 known Egyptian medical formulas are based on honey!

The Egyptians used honey combined with grease (they used vegetable oil or some snake or animal grease)—⅓ honey, ⅔ grease. Dr. Guido Manjo, in the fascinating historical text *The Healing Hand*, was surprised at this preoccupation with honey, and he decided to test its use on various types of bacteria. The honey and grease combination obliterated bacteria, and honey and butter (which has very special bacteria of its own) worked on such pathogenic bacteria as *Staphylococcus aureus*, or *E. coli*. As Dr. Manjo explains it, the grease and the honey together would prevent the bandage from sticking, and both would have a soothing effect. The obvious aspect of honey's healing abilities must be its water-drawing (hypertonic) effect, "as it draws water from the bacterial cells and causes them to shrivel and die. This mechanism works so well that an offering of honey, piously buried in Paestum in a sacred chamber 2500 years ago, never decayed, and is recognizable to this day."

Dr. Manjo is an internationally known pathologist and historical scholar, and it is to him I owe another interesting scientific explanation of the antibiotic abilities of honey, active in dilutions as low as 13 percent. The bees secrete an enzyme in which one of the active principles is inhibine. This breaks down chemically to produce H_2O_2 which is hydrogen peroxide, a common household disinfectant (which is almost identical with a mild antibiotic). Inhibine is destroyed by light and heat, and thus it is very worthwhile to obtain honey extracted only by centrifugal force and no heating or "cooking." During war shortages, honey was often used, with oil or lard, as a dressing for small wounds or ulcers, and was so used in Shanghai during World War II.

Antifatigue ★   The simple sugars in honey are immediately absorbed by the body; thus, if you need an immediate lift, add honey to some herbal tea, or add some honey to water and drink it. Early Olympic athletes used honey in great quantities before the games, and often long-distance swimmers, runners, or mountain climbers do the same in preparation for an event. The RAF pilots working almost twenty-four-hour-a-day missions during the Battle of Britain in World War II also were given enormous quantities of honey and water to increase their capacity to work.

Apple cider vinegar and honey plus some water has been used for thousands of years by several different cultures as an almost perfect balancing, or rebalancing, "food." It is not only very useful in overcoming fatigue, but this combination (use 1 teaspoon to 1 tablespoon of each to a glass of water), tastes delicious, and may be helpful in overcoming some types of arthritic deposits.

Arthritis Deposits ★   We came across the combination of apple cider vinegar and honey when a friend of ours developed a "touch" of gout. We helped him to investigate possible natural cures. Very soon after he started to take apple cider vinegar and honey, he felt better each morning—that is to say he felt really energetic—and before long he was not troubled by the gout pain. Years later he was X-rayed again, and the deposits had disappeared.

My husband, who works in film and theater and is also a professor at a university, advised one of his film crew friends about this preparation. This gaffer (the head electrician on a film) was almost crippled with arthritic nodules on his hands, and he was having a tough time working. After not seeing him for several years, my husband met him and was astonished at the change in his old friend, who looked taller and had more color. His hands were straight and supple. "Look at my hands," the gaffer demanded of my husband. "This is due to you. I've been taking your apple cider vinegar and honey and water every day—and the darn knots and the pain have disappeared! Say—I guess I should have called you to thank you!"

Honey Ointment   An ointment is a salve mixed with some plant substance and grease. I find that honey is almost a perfect "as is" ointment, and in emergencies, especially those involved with sores in the mouth or the vagina, honey is a quick, almost perfect healer.

For a more complicated ointment, add together a teaspoon each of wheat germ oil, comfrey root—or comfrey leaf—tea, and honey, and heat the mixture in the top part of a double boiler to thoroughly combine the ingredients.

In Europe, honey ointments were often made by combining a little flour and honey.

Honey Wine   Honey combined with water can produce the fermented substance called mead. It not only is intoxicating but very energizing, and was used by all the northern and western tribes of Europe in enormous quantities. While each country had different recipes and rituals connected with this simple drink, it usually was honey and water and some spices. You can use wooden kegs, stoneware kegs, or even glass bottles (in an emergency) to make this drink.

Simple Mead

1   cup (or 1 part) honey
3   cups (or 3 parts) water

Simmer the honey and water together slowly. Allow one cup of the water to evaporate. Strain off the top surface, and put the remaining liquid into a stoneware crock or dark bottle. Put a towel over it so that it will breathe, yet be free of dirt. Place it in a cool place. You can add cinnamon, cloves, or the juice of one-half lemon if you like.

Larger Quantity Honey Wine (Mead)

2   pounds honey
3   quarts water (apple juice can also be used in part)
3   small pieces or 1 large piece bark cinnamon
3   cloves
     juice of 2 or 3 lemons. Peel of 1 lemon (scrubbed)
1   teaspoon activated yeast
     crock large enough for mead to expand

Simmer the honey, water (or apple juice and water), cinnamon, cloves, and lemon juice for thirty minutes. Strain the liquid and pour it into a large earthenware crock. Do not fill the crock to the top, so as to allow an expansion of the liquid. After the mixture has cooled, add the yeast, cover the crock with a towel, and store it in a cool place (55 degrees F.) for thirty days or so. Stir from time to time.

Honey Water   Honey water (the Greeks had a name for it: *hydromel*) is the simple mixture of honey with water. Simmer a cup of water and a teaspoon of honey for five minutes. This can be added to tea, drunk alone, or used as an eye lotion. Dip the cloth in the honey-saturated water, and apply it to the closed eye. This preparation was used by the many ancient herbalists, and the nineteenth-century herbalist, Father Kneipp, recommended it highly.

Honey Gargle   The very thought of honey's soothing abilities can almost eliminate a sore throat or a chest cough. Certainly it is one of the prime aids for any respiratory problem. You can easily overcome a possible cold by drinking sage, peppermint, or chamomile tea laced with lots and lots of good honey. This honey and water can be cooled and used as a gargle, too.

Another wonderful honey remedy is to mix honey with hot lemonade and just drink away a cough! It acts so quickly and pleasantly, it certainly won't feel like medicine at all.

Still another honey gargle is a mixture of a tablespoon of honey and apple cider vinegar added to a cup of water. Drink it or gargle with it.

Honey as a Cosmetic ★   Because honey attracts and retains fluids, it is a useful ingredient in retaining moisture on the face, and it acts like a moisturizer. Honey is an excellent addition to other facial ingredients such as clay, oil, egg (whole or yolk), ground nuts, nut oils, vegetable oils, or powdered brewer's yeast. Use between a teaspoon to a tablespoon of the honey—it will help to combine other runny materials and help them to stick to the face.

Honey alone, honey added to rosewater, or with colloidal oatmeal or leftover breakfast oatmeal may be used for chapped skin or to restore dry skin to normal. Combine it with avocado or apricot oil, or your favorite home vegetable oil.

Cooking with Honey   Most of us want to substitute a good honey for the sugar in recipes, but honey is not quite as predictable as sugar in baking. Lighter colors and flavors seem to work better in baking, but I actually prefer the darker honeys for home tea, and especially for the herbal tea used to

offset respiratory problems, but this is only a personal prefer-
ence.

On the whole, when you substitute honey for sugar you
have to use less liquid by the cup. Always *deduct* three
tablespoons of any other liquid in the recipe for every cup of
honey you use. If the recipe calls for one cup of dry sugar, use
only two-thirds cup of honey, or—if you can weigh the
materials—a pound of sugar means you need to use a pound
of honey. Craig Claiborne of *The New York Times* suggests these
proportions: for 1 cup of sugar, substitute ¾ cup plus one
tablespoon (13 tablespoons all together) of honey.

Also, in making jams or jellies with honey, do it in small
batches; it will work out better. I find that for jams it is best to
use the honey by weight. Use equal amounts of fruit to honey
but discard ¼ cup liquid for every pound of honey used. The
product Sure-Jell works well.

Children   Some uncooked honeys may contain botulism or-
ganisms. These are easily digested and eliminated by adults,
according to the Center for Disease Control in Atlanta, but can
cause terrible diarrhea in the immature digestive system of
infants up to one year of age. For this reason, the Center
advises all parents to forgo using honey as a food for the infant
until the child is one year of age.

THYME
(Thymus vulgaris)

For Women   Every New Year from now on, as you fleetingly
think of Father Time, I want you also to think of the ancients'
"Mother" Thyme. The leaves of this lovely aromatic wild,
garden, and window-sill plant, now mainly known for culinary flavoring of stews, soups, and stuffings, was once considered an important herbal medicine. Because it was so effective
in overcoming uterine problems, it was often called "mother."
The leaves and flowering tops can be added to boiling water

and steeped to create a sweet, fragrant, yet slightly camphoraceous, almost bitter tea. Don't be put off by the unusual aroma and flavor, for the tea is antiseptic and healing. Even honey made from thyme plants is healing, particularly for coughs and sore throats.

Kunzle   In some ways the nineteenth-century Swiss herbalist Kunzle has put this herb into his own "thyme" capsule with this brief summary:

> Thyme is a low, creeping and lawn-forming weed, with little reddish blossoms and an intense, pleasant smell. Used as a tea (only infused), it will refresh the lungs, remove indigestion, flatulence, liver and splenetic complaints, act as a diuretic. Weakly children will be strengthened by Thyme baths. The Mountain Thyme is to be found in great quantities in sunny, dry spots. Bees and bumblebees know it, bugs and vermin avoid it.

With Other Herbs   Here is an interesting fact about thyme: It is more effective when used with other herbs. So if you feel the need of perspiration to overcome a budding cold, add thyme to any combination of herbs you might already use as a cold remedy. I would like to suggest, in particular, peppermint with either elderflower and yarrow, or a pinch of ginseng, or a dash of cayenne.

Range of Use ★   The tea has a wide range of medicinal uses and may be quite beneficial in overcoming gastric problems of wind, colic, and even bad breath. (This is usually from bad digestion, if it isn't from decayed teeth.) Gerard liked to use thyme for digestive problems, and suggested boiling wild thyme in wine "against the wamblings and gripings of the belly." Culpeper also claimed that it is a comfort for the stomach. Thyme is also an antiseptic, a first aid, allays fever, is useful for headache, and is a great insect repellent.

Whooping Cough Whooping cough was an enormous problem when I was a child, and I recall my mother and father making up syrups of thyme and honey during one siege. Today I came across a comment from a Finnish journal describing just this attribute of thyme in fighting whooping cough. The Finnish physician-author states that fresh thyme tea, using between an ounce and a half to possibly six ounces of the herb a day, plus honey, is a helpful treatment of the disease. Fortunately, most youngsters are now vaccinated against whooping cough.

Sore Throat Thyme tea laced with honey is also often effective in fighting sore throat and post nasal drip. Use a tablespoon several times a day.

Lungs Thyme tea is a reliable folk medicine for the elimination of phlegm, and is helpful in overcoming shortness of breath. Culpeper says, "It is so harmless, you need not fear the use of it."

Fever Last winter one of the students in my herbal-medicine class was visiting friends when she discovered that her three-year-old had a high fever. She looked for some herbs in her friend's cupboard and couldn't find anything but poultry seasoning (it had thyme, marjoram, and the like). She made a tea of the seasoning, gave it cold (cold for children's bronchial involvement, please), zipped the child into a sleeping bag, and let him sweat it out. He was fine in a few hours.

Since thyme is even better, medicinally, when mixed with other herbs, for adults add a pinch of ginseng in the case of bad coughing, and such soothing and emollient herbs as marshmallow root tea, slippery elm powder (or tablets), or the slightly butterscotch-smelling fenugreek, or comfrey root or leaf tea.

Headache Used cold, thyme can relieve a headache. When thyme tea is taken hot, it is said to be a central nervous system relaxer and, thus, has a folk reputation for warding off nightmares.

First Aid Since thyme is available in almost any store, it can be used liberally as a first-aid poultice. Make up a paste of moist (hot-moistened) thyme leaves and apply it to the skin to relieve the pain of an abscess, boil, or swelling. A hot poultice of thyme can help to relieve the pain of a sciatic attack, too. The oil from thyme—thymol—is sometimes used for rheumatic pains and can act like an anesthetic on the skin. Since there is always a possibility of a skin reaction with a strong oil, use cautiously, or combine with olive oil.

Antiseptic (See mention of thyme under "Antiseptic.") M. Grieve, the author of *A Modern Herbal*, notes "Thymol (oil of thyme) is a powerful antiseptic for both internal and external use; it is also employed as a deodorant and local anaesthetic. It is extensively used to medicate gauze and wool for surgical dressings. It resembles carbolic acid in its action, but is less an irritant to wounds, while its germicidal action is greater. It is, therefore, preferable as a dressing and during recent years has been one of the most extensively used antiseptics."

A long list of the physiological uses of thymol then follows:

> as an antiseptic lotion and mouthwash; as a paint in ringworm, in exzema, psoriasis, broken chilblains, parasitic skin affections and burns; as an ointment, half-strength, perfumed with lavender, to keep off gnats and mosquitos. Thymol in oily solution is applied to the respiratory passages by means of a spray in nasal catarrh, and a spiritous solution may be inhaled for laryngitis, bronchial affections and whooping cough. It is most useful given in large doses, to robust adults; in capsules, as a vermifuge, to expel parasites, especially the miner's worm; and it has also been used in diabetes and vesical catarrh.

Some allergic people may be skin-sensitive to thymol.

Insects ★ The ability of thyme to deter insects was well known by the Greeks who actually used thyme as a fumigator. Certainly it is one of the essentials in the potpourris used for linens. I use it along with lavender in my antimoth concoctions. I make up these blends fresh every summer and I never have any trouble.

GARLIC
[Allium sativum]

If garlic wasn't so cheap we would treasure it as if it were pure gold. If you haven't tried a fresh mashed garlic bud in your luncheon and evening salad, this is the time to start. For this herb adds valuable natural cleansing, infection-fighting chemicals to the daily diet. Garlic can be made into a vinegar tincture, a several-centuries-old antiepidemic body wash; into a syrup to control asthma; into a garlic oil for internal and external use; an anti-rheumatic and anti-infection cider-garlic-horseradish drink and poultice; into a restorative garlic soup. Garlic draws out pain, helps in resisting a cold, is an aid in combating hypertension, is a remarkable vermifuge (releases worms from the system), quiets the body, tranquilizes, can be put directly on warts to whittle them down, can be used (diluted in lots of water) to irrigate the colon to control amoebic dysentery, and can help treat mild cases of mononucleosis. In other words, plain old garlic is nothing short of fantastic and its use can be traced to centuries of use among many cultures.

Bacterial Infection ★ While garlic has only 1 percent of the impact of penicillin, it is nevertheless more effective with gram negative bacteria than is penicillin. Besides, it sweeps through the body in a tonic and cleansing fashion that has no side effects and doesn't destroy all the body's good intestinal flora.

Onions, lemon, and garlic are three marvelous foods, and all will help you resist most bacterial infections. When you feel a cold coming, why not combine them as I do into a mouthwatering salad? Dice lots of large beefsteak tomatoes and onions (red are actually the best for this), then add many cloves of mashed garlic plus fresh lemon juice and a vegetable oil. Add a dash of cayenne, and you will unclog a stuffed nose and chase away a cold (and possibly some friends that evening).

As for colds, researchers have discovered they are sometimes self-induced; you subconsciously or consciously think you need a vacation. How much better off you will be when you truly work against the cold with baths, herbal drinks, herb foods, herb cleansers—and willpower. Then take off the day if you wish, do something you *really* want to do. When you discover you have this power, you will also find that you have a lot of energy, too.

Garlic Soup Mash and simmer 3 clusters of peeled garlic buds (about 30), and add them to any clear chicken soup or chicken bouillon. Simmer the quart of soup for about ten minutes. Strain out the garlic buds, and add two thoroughly beaten egg yolks. Simmer again to a high heat, and serve immediately.

This is a nourishing, anti-infection soup.

Antibiotic Garlic is so strong an antibiotic that the British purchased it by the ton in World War I to control wounds. They pressed the cloves, diluted the juice with water, and placed the preparation on fresh spaghnum moss, which was applied to the wound. Journals of that period note that this procedure permitted no cases of sepsis. The Russians used garlic on wounds during World War II, in the absence of other general antibiotics. It is also used as an antiflu remedy in Russia.

To draw out pain from joints, toothaches, and earaches, place the crushed raw bulb on a piece of *gauze* (otherwise some of these strong herbs can cause blisters on delicate skin) and place the gauze over the area of pain. For the joints, use a garlic paste. For the ear, use slivers, in *gauze*. I recall how when I was a young child my father cured my friend's terrible and persistent earache with this simple cure. This ear cure took about a week. An infection in the lobe will often take three days to a week. Naturally, garlic cures take longer than swift-acting antibiotics which, however, your physician may consider preferable.

Abscess   We lived in the country every summer and had some interesting connections with some "hill folk." One spring Billy-Bob came down to see "Doc" (my father), and showed him his inflamed and dangerously abscessed leg. "They tell me they can't help me with this in the hospital, Doc, and they say it might have to come off. Can you help me?" Dad took down two whole clusters of garlic (we always had them hanging on a string in the kitchen) and mashed about thirty buds into a paste. He placed the paste on a gauze right over the infection and covered the paste with a warm flannel bandage.

Two days later Dad took off the bandage (it had an incredible smell). He washed the wound with calendula lotion and sage tea and then replaced a fresh, clean garlic-paste poultice. This was allowed to stay for several days, and when this came off, the wound was ready for another series of washings with diluted calendula tincture and some peach-pit tea. Then Dad made a fresh goldenseal, plantain, and comfrey ointment and packed the wound. Billy-Bob never ever had trouble with that infection and was forever grateful.

Cider Anti-Infection Wash, Rheumatism Liniment ★

    1   quart apple cider
    4   ounces garlic juice
    ½   ounce grated horseradish root

Add garlic and horseradish to the cider. Place the cider in a warm place for twelve hours. Shake the container often. Then remove it to a cool place. Let is stand another twelve hours. Strain the liquid and place it in a labeled jar. Keep it in a cool place or refrigerator.

To fight infection, use this preparation, a teaspoon at a time, internally, one to three times a day between meals, or externally on a cloth for a wound or painful joints. This is a stimulating wash for rheumatic, sciatic, or arthritic pain, and can be used to encourage circulation in some paralyzed parts. For sensitive skin first apply an oil such as castor oil.

Vinegar of the Four Thieves (see Section Three: How to Make the Herbal Medicine) ★   This is a vinegar wash used to deter disease-bearing insects during epidemics. It can be used to cleanse a sickroom and to prevent the spread of certain bacterial infections, especially in close quarters like dormitories, schools, an army, or cooperative communities.

Teeth   Because garlic acts almost like an antibiotic, friends have used it to draw the infection from abscessed teeth. However, mouth abscesses are dangerous and can cause complications. See a physician as soon as possible.

Pain   Garlic, like other sharp juice roots and bulbs—onions, masterwort, and new potatoes—draws out pain. Mashed garlic, garlic oil, or garlic tincture can be used with excellent effect on wounds, abscesses, or pus-forming infections. However, it is strong, and may cause a blister on surrounding tissue.

Enema   The garlic enema is one of the many remarkable cleansers in the herbal world. We have traveled in Mexico where there is a great deal of amoebic dysentery, and we once lived with a group of people who came down with it. Those who used blended fresh garlic-and-water enemas felt fine in a few days. Some friends who live on a commune had an epidemic of mononucleosis. Those who were willing to take water-and-garlic enemas restored their energy in a comparatively short time. Others took months to recover. Only a few garlic buds are needed. Crush, blend with a quart of water.

Vermifuge ★   Almost every folk medicine notes the use of garlic juice, garlic in salads, garlic pearls, garlic oil, or garlic sandwiches to cleanse the entire system internally and help make the blood healthy while eliminating any poisonous bacteria, toxins, or worms. Garlic oil, in particular, is very successful folk medicine in eliminating pin worms and thread worms from the body. To find out if you have worms (rectal itching is frequently one sign), attach Scotch tape in the rectal fissure—it will "catch" the worms like fly paper. This does not cure the condition however; it is only a diagnostic tool. There are many herbal worm cures; check them all out.

Garlic Oil   To make garlic oil, which can be used in small amounts on salads or saved for medicinal purposes, blend one cup of peeled garlic buds and one cup of olive oil in a labeled jar, and then add a cup of olive oil. Let the garlic be absorbed into the oil for a week, but shake the jar several times a day. Strain out the garlic, and keep the liquid cold in the refrigerator. We have used this oil externally on wounds for adults, internally, or in salads, especially when swift cleansing action and antibacterial action is needed. A few drops of the oil can often help with low-grade body infections.

Garlic Syrup for Asthma   My dad's family treasured this unique folk remedy to control asthma attacks and it may be of some value to many of you when you are unable to get to your physician. The dose is 1 teaspoon with, or without, water every fifteen minutes until the asthma spasm is controlled. Afterwards give the patient one teaspoon every two to three hours for the rest of the day. Following the crest of the attack, give one teaspoon three times a day.

> ½   pound peeled garlic buds
> equal amounts vinegar and distilled water
> (enough to cover garlic buds)
> ½   pint glycerine
> 1½ pounds honey

Peel the garlic. Add equal amounts of vinegar and distilled water to cover the garlic. Use a wide-mouth jar; close it tightly,

and shake well. Stand it in a cool place for four days. Shake it
once or twice a day.

Add the glycerine. Shake the jar and let it stand another
day. Strain the liquid with pressure through a sieve. Blend in
the honey, and place the liquid in a labeled jar. Store in a cool
place.

Optional: Simmer three ounces of fennel seeds, and/or
caraway seeds for half an hour and add it to the mixture while
it is steeping and before it is strained.

Hypertension   According to folk medicine, as well as many
recent laboratory experiments, garlic has the unique ability to
bring down high blood pressure. As a preventive use garlic
tea, or garlic oil in drops, throughout the day or, if fresh garlic
is offensive, use garlic capsules. Hypertension is a serious
health problem. Be sure to consult your family physician for
diagnosis and control.

Hypoglycemia   Experiments in India were reported in *Lancet*,
the British medical journal. There is some indication that
onions and garlic may have a positive effect in diabetes.

Arteriosclerosis   The same issue of *Lancet* reported other
Indian experiments. The indications are that garlic may have
"significant protective action" and could be used for long-term
preventive use without danger of toxicity if there is a family
history of this disease.

Adult Colic   For adult spasms, combine three cloves of garlic
with five tablespoons of caraway seed, and simmer that for
about fifteen minutes in milk. Strain the liquid, add some
boiled water, and drink it.

HORSERADISH
[Cochlearia armoracia]

This root is a potent stimulant for the body, and country
wisdom indicates it may be used internally to clear the nasal

passages, reduce fluid in the system, act as a digestive aid, and cleanse the system of infection.

You can grow the root—and, frankly, the taste is far superior to the old roots found in most markets. Horseradish sauce can be purchased in the refrigerated section of any market.

To dry the fresh roots, wash, scrub, and hand dry them, and cut the long root into strips. Dry them in a low-temperature oven. Store them in labeled jars. These roots can be added to salad dressings and soups, or used as side dressings for meat or in medicinal preparations. Here are some of our many generation-old recipes.

Sinus Remedy

> juice of 1 fresh, peeled pulped horse-radish root
> juice of 2–3 lemons

Combine the two juices together. Place the liquid in a labeled jar, and store it in the refrigerator (lemon juice is susceptible to mold). Use half a teaspoon at a time between meals. Use it for several months until the mucus in the sinus area is cleared up.

A word on this remedy: It is sharp and will undoubtedly bring tears to your eyes, but this is considered an evidence of its effectiveness.

Tissue-Swelling (Edema) (For persistent water retention, see a physician.)

> 4 tablespoons freshly grated horseradish root
> 2 cups apple cider vinegar
> 4 tablespoons glycerine
> a preservative
> screw-top bottle

Add the freshly grated root to the cider. Place the cider in a warm place for half a day. Occasionally open the jar or loosen the screw top, and shake. The second part of the day, move the preparation to a cool place. Keep on shaking the jar every once in a while. After about twelve hours, strain out the horseradish. Add the glycerine. Bottle, label, and keep in a cool place.

Internal use: Drink one tablespoon several times a day. External use: Heat the liquid, and apply it on cotton or a washcloth to the swollen tissue areas.

The horseradish-apple cider-garlic drink for internal infection: See the entry for Garlic (page 65).

Horseradish Toothbrush Did you ever wonder how people washed their teeth before machine-made toothbrushes were devised? They made them from resilient twigs, such as dogwood, or from various roots, such as horseradish, marshmallow, alfalfa, and licorice.

This next recipe has a twin advantage. It produces homemade toothbrushes as well as a very pungent and effective antiseptic mouthwash. While the cloves and the tincture of myrrh are optional, they are exceptional tooth and mouth aids. You can also add a pinch of goldenseal powder, too, if there is a need to control sores in the mouth.

Toothbrush and/or Mouthwash

1 or more roots of horseradish. Cut into 6-inch strips.
1 medium bark of cinnamon
1 pint inexpensive brandy
12 to a handful of cloves—optional: place in brandy
1 teaspoon tincture of myrrh—optional: place in brandy

(If you are using the cloves and tincture of myrrh, place them in the brandy and put them aside.) Unstrip or unravel one end of each horseradish strip. Simmer the strips in water with cinnamon bark. When the root seems tender (this may take fifteen or more minutes), strain off the water and reserve the cinnamon. Add the slightly brittle horseradish to the brandy. Soak the horseradish for three hours or more.

Mouthwash: Strain off the brandy. Reserve the horseradish for drying. Add the cinnamon and cloves to the brandy, and soak them for a few more days. This mouthwash is very strong and will have to be diluted.

Toothbrushes: Place the horseradish strips on a screen with circulating air, or in a warm oven to dry. To use, dip them in warm water and rub the gums and the teeth.

Note: In the past, these roots were dried and then soaked in one of the gum resins to harden, and dried again before using.

Old Rheumatism Remedy Some of the older doctors in our family instructed their patients to swallow tiny unbruised pieces of horseradish root without chewing, and to follow this regime for a month. For chronic rheumatism, they seem to have achieved some good results with this procedure.

Acne Cure Make up a tincture in a pint of ninety-proof alcohol (or use vinegar) with several ounces of horseradish. Add a pinch of grated nutmeg and a peel of bitter orange. Or you may purchase compound spirit of horseradish at the drugstore. Apply some tincture (or spirit) to each pimple with a cotton-tipped stick.

LEMON
[Citrus limonum]

In our family we have always known that when we use lemon juice generously, this noble fruit rewards us with better digestion, heart tonification, skin cleansing, styptic response, anticold and anti-infection action, and will act as a valuable liver decongestant. The juice of the lemon is refrigerant and, when diluted with water, is a refreshing and agreeable drink during any fever or inflammation.

Digestive Aid ★ Lemon juice and water used first thing in the morning will increase digestive juices, tone up the system, and cleanse and decongest the liver. If you are constipated, drink two glasses of cold water on arising, and drink lemon juice and water afterwards. It is a fantastic purifier and health aid in regulating digestion and eliminating waste materials. Suck a thin piece of lemon dipped in salt to overcome heartburn from sweet food.

Blood Purifier ★　Drink lots of diluted lemonade (no sugar please) to try to cleanse the system of boils and to help eliminate other skin problems.

Skin Cleanser and Blackhead Eraser　Rub lemon juice on skin to try to banish blackheads and acne. Combine the juice with salt and use the paste to rub off dead skin cells on elbows and thighs. Fingernails and hands respond very well to daily lemon rinses.

Finger Sores　To alleviate pain from finger sores or finger infections, heat a lemon in the oven, cut a narrow opening in the center of the lemon, sprinkle it with common salt, and bury the finger in the opening. Repeat this until the finger is cured of pain.

Bleeding　Lemon is often a successful styptic even when ice and other styptics fail to staunch the flow of blood. While the first squeeze of lemon stings, there is prompt relief for cuts.

Colds　Squeeze the juice of a ripe lemon into the palm of the hand and gently sniff the juice into the nostrils several times. It is quite strong, but cleansing. Also, drink herbal teas laced with lots of lemon juice and honey.

Coughs　Wash the lemon. Place it uncut on its thinnest edge, in a dish of honey and a handful of cloves. Soak the lemon and the honey overnight. Cut the lemon in half, and squeeze all the juice into the honey. Drink the lemon juice and honey, or add hot water to thin it out. Use the liquid in small doses throughout the day; it is exceptionally therapeutic.

Heart　Lemon juice is said to be helpful in creating a proper fluid action in the blood. Hardening of the arteries, fragile blood vessels, badly circulating blood, distended veins, high blood pressure—all respond to a lemon cure.

Epidemic ★   Make sure to always have a lot of fresh lemons on hand during a bacterial contagion or flu season. Squeezed lemons do not hold, but lemons may be preserved (see below). Also, you might consider using a vodka tincture in small amounts for travel, or on trips in a remote area. Purchase fresh lemons, wash in liquor, and cut them with a clean and freshly boiled knife (the knife can carry the bacteria from the skin of any fruit or vegetable you use). Add them to distilled water to make a sour lemonade. This is a therapeutic, purifying drink.

Fever   Use diluted lemon juice to refresh the patient and to help reduce fever. Use either as lemonade, or add to barley water or other mild nutritive drinks.

Itching   The National Dispensatory notes that local application of lemon relieves itching of the scrotum.

Rheumatism   Some European spas use a lemon juice cure to detoxify arthritic and rheumatic patients. Traditional Chinese medicine utilizes cut lemon rubs to relieve the pain of neuralgia.

Kidney and Bladder   Lemon juice drinks have been useful in controlling some bladder and kidney infections.

Elixir ★   Turn-of-the-century German and English physicians researched the use of lemons, and in addition to their discovering that lemon juice controls scurvy, they concluded that lemons should be used every day to prolong life.

To Preserve Lemons

6   whole lemons
Freshly squeezed lemon juice (enough to cover the lemons)
½   cup coarse salt
Sterilized pint jar

These lemons will keep up to a year. They must be covered with the lemon juice and salt. To use, rinse each lemon, as it is needed, under cold running water. This recipe is useful for some areas of the world where fresh lemons are not readily available.

Wash the lemons in apple cider vinegar. Scrub them with a brush. Wash and rinse the lemons, then dry them. Open the lemons by partially quartering them from the top to within a half inch of the bottom. Place salt inside the lemon, then make it whole again (reshape it). Place one tablespoon of salt in the bottom of the jar. Put the lemons in the jar, and push them down. Place the rest of the salt between the lemons. Push them so that some of the juice squeezes out. Add additional lemon juice if needed, as the lemon juice must cover the lemons. There should be some air space in the jar. Seal and label it.

Each day for a month, turn the jar. Keep in a warm place. Make sure the salt and the lemon juice saturate each lemon.

PEPPERMINT ★
[Mentha piperita]

This is a favorite beverage tea all over the world. It has a great many health uses. Peppermint has a strong effect on the digestive system and will help control diarrhea, spasms, and relieve indigestion. For this reason I always carry some peppermint tea and a vial of peppermint oil on my foreign travels. (See also the "Trip Insurance" section.)

Digestive Aid   Chamomile and peppermint are used in most of the spas in Europe as a digestive aid and as a switch from the disastrous effects of caffeine in coffee. While I have used it on a more or less continuous basis for many years, and I know many strong and well people who use peppermint every day, I have come to the conclusion that herbal teas should be used by mood, need, and meal and that all such teas should be interchanged for variety and effect. Since peppermint is so rich in tannin, vary your herbal beverages with other herbal blends.

Headache Aid   A drink of peppermint tea is instantly refreshing and will dispel many headaches, especially those emanating from the digestive system.

Muscle Spasms, Muscle Cramps   Drink peppermint tea to overcome muscle spasms and cramps. Also apply it externally as a wet mash to the area of the pain. The camphorous principles in peppermint will help to relieve pain.

Sinus   Drink lots of peppermint tea, and apply a large, warm peppermint pack to the sinus area. It is usually quite effective.

Important

Please refer to the Special Notice to the Reader on page *xx* and the instructions on page 117.

SOME OTHER FAVORITE HERBS IN BRIEF

(This list includes my favorite herbs.)

Alfalfa ★

Alfalfa is available in tablet, tea, or seed form. The seeds are easily sprouted and contain many minerals, some protein, and have the virtue of being crunchy as well as detoxifying. Some health-food stores carry fresh alfalfa sprouts in their refrigerator section. I sprout alfalfa together with mung beans, as they both take three days. They are a filling diet snack.

To sprout seeds, first soak them for a few hours. Drain them and place them either in a glass jar with a mesh-strainer top or, as I prefer, in a closed-top unglazed clay sprouter dish, which stands in a glass pie plate in a half inch of water. Wash and drain the sprouts once a day. In three days they will be crunchy and long enough to eat. If you want them to be green, you can place them in a jar in the sun for a day. Sprouting is not only fun kitchen gardening, but a valuable nutritional aid.

Almonds (Sweet) ★

Almonds have been used for centuries to heal the body internally and may be used ground in water against fever, chest coughs, and for nutrition. Ten almonds are the equivalent of half a pound of meat. To prepare an almond drink, grind six tablespoons of almonds in a food processor, nut grinder, or a mortar and pestle. Add a pint of cold water. This milky drink is well tolerated by invalids and may be helpful in overcoming a bronchial attack.

Aloe vera ★

This remarkable succulent may be planted in your garden or, even better, grown as a house plant to be kept in the kitchen as an antiburn remedy and as a cosmetic aid. To obtain the gel, break open a leaf and smear the juice on a burn or on an insect bite to alleviate the pain. This gel will relieve many skin irritations, including sunburn, and will also soften rough skin. Recent experiments indicate this same gel is successful in alleviating the pain of rheumatic joints. Aloe vera gel can be purchased in many health-food stores.

Angelica [Angelica archangelica]

Angelica tea, which is useful for delayed menstrual period and to overcome the effects of stomach gas, is prepared by simmering one ounce of the clean root in a pint of water. Use garden angelica if you want to candy the stalks, as they do in France and Spain; wild angelica flowers look a lot like poison hemlock flowers, so don't pick them unless you know the difference!

Anise [Pimpinella anisum]

Anise tea is an excellent aid for children's flatulence, and since the seeds contain a strong oil (anethol) which has a beneficial effect on bronchial tubes, it can be used for upper respiratory problems. An effective shortcut is to use the liqueur, anisette, added to hot water, to overcome nausea, sluggish digestion, and especially to help during bronchitis or a bronchial asthma attack. Anise oil is useful in destroying lice and itching insects.

Apple ★

"To eat an apple going to bed/Will make the doctor beg his bread." Apples are easily digested and contain solvents, stabilizers, muscle builders, brain and body builders, oxygen carriers, and bone builders in the form of various minerals.

The fruit sugar from the apple is readily available and quickly passes into the bloodstream. The malic and tartaric acid in the apple neutralize any overacidity in the body. That is why apples are often used in monofasts to detoxify the body, overcome digestive problems, and help with gout. Eat sweet apples if you have too much acid in the system. Eat sour apples if you have too little acid, and/or are constipated.

Apples are a great tooth cleanser.

Apples are fine first aid. Use them raw, peeled and grated as a poultice, or roast the apple in an oven and extract the pulp. Use this pulp on the eyes to relieve any kind of strain or inflammation. Overripe apples are used in some parts of England to relieve rheumatic and weak eyes. Raw, overripe, or roasted apple pulp can be used to good effect as a poultice on any type of sprain.

Apple water is a good cooling drink for fever. In American pioneer medicine, apple bark decoction was used to bring down high fevers.

Vinegar made from apples has many medicinal and health uses. Apple cider vinegar is an excellent cosmetic aid and can be mixed with rosewater for a daily restorative face splash. Use a cup of apple cider vinegar in a bath to soften the skin and to help reduce fatigue.

Arnica (See *My Favorite Herbs.*)

Asparagus

The water from steamed asparagus and asparagus stalks is diuretic. In the past, Dr. S. J. Jefferson of England prescribed an asparagus tincture to be used in half-teaspoon doses along with other herbal diuretics. To make this tincture: Express the juice from five pounds of fresh asparagus. Simmer it until it reduces to a pint. Strain it and add to a pint of ninety-proof spirit. Instead of fresh stalks, five ounces of dried tops of asparagus may be used to prepare the tincture.

Balm *(Folia melissae)*

"The juice of the Balm glueth together green wounds," says Gerard, and, as did many ancient herbalists, he noted the pain-deadening properties of this plant. European herbalists often use balm in the bath to overcome neuralgic of spasmatic pain.

Drink hot balm tea to induce perspiration for detoxification purposes or add balm to peppermint, elderflower, ginger, or other such antirespiratory herbal teas.

Cold balm, in fresh form, is best for wounds as the balsamic oil needed for cuts and bruises is dispelled by heating. Use cold balm tea infused in cold water for children's flatulence, too, and to calm the nerves or overcome nervous headache. Incidentally, lavender, peppermint, and benzoin (a resin) also contain similar balsamic oils.

Barley (Pearl Barley)
[Hordeum distichon]

Barley is an ancient cereal grain and has long been used by physicians to add nutrition to an invalid's diet, to aid in fever reduction, and to control infant diarrhea. (See Barley Water in Section 3.) To overcome extreme bladder and urinary passage irritation, prepare this ancient remedy: Add cooked barley to one ounce of dissolved gum arabic (you can also use the gelatin of Irish moss or agar-agar), and two glasses of boiling water. Stir, and drink when cool.

Basil (Sweet)
[Ocymum basilicum]

The bruised leaves of sweet basil give off a delightful aroma. Pour one cup of boiling water over two tablespoons of the garden leaves for a mild and effective tea said to relieve delayed menstruation. Basil will relieve the pain of insect stings, and may be added to insect-repellent preparations.

Beets

This exceptional vegetable can be used fresh, juiced, or purchased as an organic powder or tablet. It is a powerful liver and body cleanser and can be used to help overcome many blood problems. It is also a great tonic. Since concentrated beets are very potent, first start with a small amount and gradually work up to larger amounts. Some students have reported back to me on the use of beet juice or pills to regulate their irregular menstrual periods, and the results were usually excellent.

Use beet juice combined with carrot juice as a blood builder for anemia; this is reported to also help lower the body cholesterol.

If you have a juicer, don't throw away those marvelous and mineral-rich beet tops. Juice them, add some watercress, and sweeten the drink with a can of pineapple juice.

Bilberry (or Blueberry)
[Vaccinium myrtillus]

Blueberry or bilberry (or huckleberry) was used and praised by ancient herbalists for the control of diarrhea or dysentery and for urinary disorders. This berry has astringent and germicidal action within the system. I pick fresh wild or garden blueberries and prepare an extract by pouring a handful into a pint of inexpensive brandy. The berries release a great deal of tannin—which is what controls the diarrhea. The dose is a tablespoon of the extract in a half glass of room-temperature water every two hours until the diarrhea stops.

A syrup of blueberries was used by ancient Greek herbalists to control the flow of mother's milk.

Use the extract for dry eczema. Paint the scales with the extract and cover them with gauze. Repeat this once a day until the eczema is controlled.

Some people with diabetes have claimed they have controlled the disease with extended use of blueberry leaf tea, so it may be worth adding to a diabetic diet.

Blackberry (See *My Favorite Herbs.*)

Cabbage

White cabbage leaves may reduce swelling, and they have an affinity for pus. Break the high ridges of the leaf, dip the leaf in warm water, and apply it as a poultice on running and infected sores. Attach the cabbage with a large, loose bandage. As soon as the leaf feels hot from the internal inflammation, replace it. Red cabbage leaves can be made into an anticough syrup or nourishing soup during any illness.

Calendula (See *My Favorite Herbs.*)

Caraway Seeds (See *My Favorite Herbs.*)

Carrot ★

I rank carrots with garlic and cayenne in my herbal arsenal of good health. The vegetable is rich in vitamins A, B, and C, and contains small amounts of E and K, as well as phosphorus, potassium, and calcium.

Carrot juice is energy! Use carrots to try to cleanse the system of various impurities, aid many eye problems, relieve most skin problems, and help overcome many glandular disturbances. Use it every day if you are trying to regulate a menstrual period.

If you have a problem with sinus or acne, or skin eruptions, or strange eye problems that may be nutritional, your vitamin A need may be higher than the national average.

I recommend a centrifugal juicer for every family; even if it isn't used every day, it is extraordinarily useful to have to use during periods of stress, fatigue, and illness of any kind. A small glass of pure carrot juice every day will be a strong health aid to any family, especially one prone to respiratory diseases.

We eat a lot of grated carrots, too, and now with the new food processors this grating is no longer a chore. Add lemon, oil, and garlic to this nutritious salad and serve it once or twice a week for the family.

Infant Diarrhea   Add peeled (if nonorganic source) carrots to every soup. Carrot soup is an unsurpassed home remedy for infant diarrhea. It works by preventing the severe loss of body fluid and by supplying water to overcome dehydration. Cooked carrots are high in potassium (this mineral is needed during any illness), phosphorus, and sodium, and also contain pectin, a valuable antidiarrhea aid. The cooked carrots in soup coat the inflamed small bowel, soothe it, and thus promote healing. The soup increases peristalsis, slows down any diarrhea-creating bacteria growth, and also overcomes the need to vomit. Use carrot soup for an entire week, and meanwhile, as soon as the infant seems ready for additional food, you can add boiled rediluted skim milk and ripe or dried pectin-rich bananas to the diet.

Poultice   For a healing and antiseptic poultice for use on cuts, wounds, abscesses, and inflammations, use either raw, grated carrots or cooked, mashed carrots.

Powder as Universal Remedy ★   Another exceptional and fairly little known way to use carrots is in the dried state. Grate carrots into the tiniest pieces, and dry them on white paper or in your home food dryer. (You can rig up your own in a large wooden box with shelves and one or two low-wattage light bulbs.) This concentrates the useful vitamins and minerals contained in the carrot. Store this material in a dark, labeled jar. These carrots can be added to soups to restore body energy, or used in a capsule or in pill form (add to scrambled eggs or roll in cream cheese) as a potent remedy to overcome infection, glandular disturbances, headaches, or joint problems. In fact, whenever you feel unwell add some of these dried carrots to your other foods, herbal drinks, vegetable juices, or soups. It has strong healing abilities. This is good, cheap, and effective medicine.

Catnip

Use catnip tea compresses on the forehead to release pressure from the eyes and overcome a headache. The tea will also relieve the pain of bee stings.

Cayenne (See *My Favorite Herbs.*)

Celandine (Greater Celandine)
[Chelidonium majus] ★

I first learned about this herb from a Latvian nurse. This herb, which grows inconspicuously in our wastelands, has a small, brilliant yellow blossom, and the stem exudes a vivid yellow juice when cut or bruised. A tincture of this herb made from the entire plant is considered a virtual panacea by some peoples of Eastern Europe. They use eight to ten drops of the tincture steeped in brandy or ninety-proof spirit—or eight to ten drops of the fresh expressed juice—three times a day to overcome sluggish liver, for neuralgia of the face and head, or neuralgia of the shoulder, especially on the right side of the body. It is also useful when there is a thick urine, or clay-like stools and constipation. The prepared tincture is available from many pharmacies with European clientele. Use in moderation and for limited time periods.

The juice of the living plant is also a great wound remedy to allay pain (celandine is a member of the poppy family) and is an old and effective wart remedy.

Centuary *[Erythraea centaurium]*

Use the flowers and tops of this garden plant and infuse them in cold water for several hours to prepare a drink that

will remedy many stomach problems, particularly heartburn.
A hot tea will often help overcome pain of muscular rheumatism.

Chamomile (See *My Favorite Herbs*.)

Cherry (Wild) *[Prunus serotina]*

Wild cherry bark is still in the official pharmacopoeia and
is thus available, in syrup form, to overcome colds and
irritating coughs from bronchitis. Use a teaspoon of the syrup
in 2 tablespoons of water every three hours (adult dose).
Collect the bark fresh each season because it deteriorates
quickly. It has the odor of almonds which almost disappears,
but which emerges again when the bark is powdered. See
syrup recipe or release the bark in alcohol or water, but do not
boil it, as heat destroys its medicinal value.

Chickweed (See *My Favorite Herbs*.)

Chicory (See *My Favorite Herbs*.)

Cloves (See *My Favorite Herbs*.)

Coltsfoot *[Tussilago farfara]*

Since ancient Greek times the leaf of the gay yellow-
flowered coltsfoot has been associated with chest complaints.
It is used in a very special way: Either make up an infusion
with licorice sticks and honey, and drink the tea, or powder
the dried leaves and smoke them! Coltsfoot has always been
an important ingredient in British herbal tobacco and may be
used alone or mixed with small amounts of thyme, lavender,
chamomile, eyebright, buckbean, or betony for pipe tobacco.

The smoke may also be directed to the nostrils or mouth through a funnel and has been said to be an aid in overcoming difficult breathing, bronchitis, or asthma attacks.

Warm water added to the dried leaves will make a soothing poultice for inflamed or rough skin.

Comfrey (See *My Favorite Herbs.)*

Coriander *[Coriandrum sativum]*

Fresh coriander and coriander seeds are available for cooking purposes and in fresh form for interesting flavor additions to Mexican, Indian, and Chinese food. I am indebted to Craig Claiborne of *The New York Times* for his special way of storing fresh coriander (which is available with roots intact from Chinese groceries): "I insert the roots and the stems—up to the mid-section—in cold water. I then place a loose-fitting plastic bag over the leaves, allowing space for air around the bottom of the bag. I find that the leaves will stay green, fresh and unblemished for up to ten days, depending on the freshness of the coriander when purchased."

The herb was first used by the Romans as a spice, and then as a remedy for chills and fever, and is a help in warming the stomach and overcoming flatulence. Its Latin name means "bug," and frankly it does smell a bit musty, but when it is dry it has a most pleasant odor. Despite its strange smell, this is the most commonly used flavoring herb in the world.

Honey of Coriander ★ This honey will stimulate digestion and appetite and is said to be almost magical in banishing flatulence and internal gas from the system. It also sweetens the breath. Mix this honey with any herb that may cause griping or cramps, as when using a strong herbal cathartic like senna. To make this honey, combine oil of coriander, which should be available in the drugstore, add honey, and mix while both are warm.

Curry Powder   This curry powder can be used in many ways, including as a marinade with yogurt for roast chicken. Curries are used in very hot climates to stimulate the system and maintain inner vitality and are, therefore, very useful during a hot summer.

1   ounce coriander seed powder
1   ounce ginger root powder
1   ounce cardamom seed powder
3   ounces turmeric powder
¼   ounce cayenne pepper powder

Cranberry ★

Cranberries can help fight infection. Cranberry juice is very effective as a drink and a douche in cystitis. Since cranberries are fairly high in vitamin C (a cup contains 15 milligrams), use cranberries for bleeding gums.

Cranberries contain an ingredient similar to that of the drugs that help control asthma attacks, and the following cranberry drink may help dilate the bronchial tubes.

Asthma Cranberry Drink   Fill a stainless steel, ceramic, or cast-iron pot half full of fresh washed cranberries. Fill the pot with pure filtered or distilled water. Simmer it slowly on low heat. The water will recede to the top level of the cranberries. Pour off the cooking water, strain the berries, and throw away the skins. Place the cranberry juice pulp in a labeled jar in the refrigerator. Use a teaspoon or two of the pulp in a cup of warm water to overcome an asthma attack. A few sips of this elixir may help restore normal breathing.

Dandelion (See *My Favorite Herbs.*)

Dill

Dill, which comes from the Saxon word meaning "to lull," actually has many tranquilizing abilities. For this purpose, and to help overcome hardened bowel movements, simmer a teaspoon of the bruised fruit—which we always call seed—in a cup of boiling water, strain, and place the hot seeds in bread for eating, or use the strained tea to overcome colic and wind in infants. It also increases the milk of nursing mothers.

Elderflowers and Elderberries
[Sambucus nigra] ★

Elder is one of the most versatile and effective of the herbal health aids. Both the flowers and the berries may be scalded in a hot drink and used to promote perspiration, which is useful in aborting a cold, or in respiratory problems and fever. I usually combine several tablespoons of elderflowers and a pinch of yarrow with well over half peppermint leaves. Each herb has a special function in overcoming a negative health situation.

Hemorrhoids For relief of hemorrhoids try combining the flowers of elder and honeysuckle. Pour boiling water or hot milk over the flowers, and steep them for fifteen minutes. Strain. Add additional milk or boiling water, and plunge a folded cloth into the liquid and apply the cloth piping hot to the area of pain. The green berries or leaves can also be used in an ointment for this same problem. Apply the ointment while hot.

A jelly made of the berries will cure constipation in children. The root, however, is a strong purgative, and should *only* be used by very knowledgeable herbalists.

Elecampane [Inula Helenium]

The root of this stunning yellow flower contains a powerful antiseptic called helenin. Chemically it resembles camphor. To make a tea simmer an ounce of the root in a pint of water for ten minutes. Cool. To help regulate menstruation and to overcome the effects of an obstinate old cough, use one to two tablespoons several times a day. Elecampane root was once made into lozenges to help overcome coughs.

Eyebright *[Euphrasia officinalis]* ★

Use the whole herb to strengthen the eyes. It can be made into a tea or used as the ancient herbalists did, boiled in wine and sipped at bedtime. Sebastian Kneipp recommends an infusion of strained eyebright as an eye wash, or added to home apple cider, to sip, to strengthen the stomach. For simple inflammation of the eyes, use fifteen drops of the tincture in a ¼ cup of rose water, and apply it as a compress. Replace the compress with a fresh one, and repeat this several times a day.

Fennel *[Fœniculum vulgare]*

Use bruised fennel seed in food or with caraway and anise seeds to overcome even the most obstinate attacks of gas. Make a hot tea by pouring two cups of boiling water over a teaspoon of bruised seeds. Regular drinking of fennel tea is an old folk remedy used to regulate difficult and irregular menstrual periods. Use the tea before and during the period up to three times a day. Eat the seeds to increase milk while nursing.

To promote the freer flow of urine, combine fennel seeds, caraway seeds, and juniper berries.

Fennel has still another value in medicine: According to Sebastian Kneipp the tea made from bruised seeds will help detoxify the body. Use it strained in the bath or in a vaporizer to increase the release of toxic wastes. ★

Fig *[Ficus Carica]*

Eat dried figs to overcome constipation. Use of the drawing power of figs for boils goes back to very ancient times. To ripen a boil, split a fig, heat it, and place on boil. This is particularly effective with boils on the gum.

Figs may be added to water to prepare an excellent gargle or sore throat aid. Use four tablespoons of figs to a cup of water, boil, strain, cool, and drink the liquid or use it as gargle.

Flaxseed [Linum usitatissimum]

Flaxseed contains a remarkable healing oil which can be used both externally and internally. Used externally, it is a very healing poultice for sprains, some simple growths, or combined with lime water for overcoming the pain of burns. For the poultice, release the linseed oil in the outer skin of the flaxseed with a brief soak in boiling water. Apply the whole as a mash in a clean folded cloth. Attach the cloth to the area of the sprain or pain, and replace as often as desired.

As far back as Hippocrates, flaxseed (also called linseed) tea has been used to overcome the constriction of a sore throat and hoarseness, or to calm the chest during bronchitis. The tea has soothing properties, is mildly laxative, and is useful to induce kidney activity and to soothe the pain of kidney colic and cramps. To use flaxseed as a tea, first strain 2 ounces of flaxseed in cold water. After running cold water through, place the seeds in a nonaluminum pot with 4 cups of cold water, and add a washed, thinly peeled rind of half a lemon. Simmer the liquid for about fifteen minutes on a slow fire. Strain away the seeds and add the juice of a whole lemon and a teaspoon of honey.

Do not use hardware store "boiled" linseed oil!

Garlic (See My Favorite Herbs.)

Ginger (See My Favorite Herbs.)

Ginseng (See My Favorite Herbs.)

Goldenrod [Solidago virgaurea] ★

There are many varieties of this attractive yellow flower dotting the countryside side by side with purple loosestrife during the late summer and early fall months. My grandmother advised people who were allergic to goldenrod to drink a tea made of equal parts of goldenrod flowers and juniper berries. Steep this tea, strain, and drink teaspoon doses each day for several weeks before the allergic response is anticipated. This combination of juniper and goldenrod is also used by some of my favorite Swiss herbalists to relieve kidney and bladder inflammation and to overcome sleeplessness. For these problems, use a teaspoon of each of the herbs to every cup of boiling water. Drink half a cup three to five times a day. If possible, consult your physician before undertaking this regime, however.

Goldenseal [Hydrastis canadensis]

This is a fascinating and useful, almost cure-all, herb, much admired by the American Indians, pioneers through the West, and by early naturopaths. Small amounts can be ingested as a tea and will have a profound effect on many organs. Large amounts of this potent golden powder cleanse the system so fast that I consider large amounts to be toxic. Be very conservative in dealings with plants—have great respect for their power. I, myself, therefore, prefer to use goldenseal externally on the whole, except in the mouth, where I combine it with tincture of myrrh. It is a very strong antiseptic, disinfectant, and astringent. Internally, it is *not* indicated for pregnant women (or at least it can be used only in very tiny amounts), for hypoglycemics, or people with hypertension. When there is a doubt about certain uses of an herb, *don't take chances*—there are plenty of other herbs.

External Use   For sore gums, use your fingers or a toothbrush to paint the gums with goldenseal powder, or combine the powder and a few drops of tincture of myrrh—an extremely effective combination for any mouth problem, even pyorrhea.

Mouth Sores   Use a cotton-tipped stick to place the powder directly on a cold sore or canker sore. It will help to relieve the pain and will usually control the situation overnight. If you prefer, you can gargle constantly with the powder or tincture of myrrh and water, but use a strong solution.

Tooth Extraction   Apply the goldenseal root powder directly on the wound to heal it, and chomp on a comfrey root or comfrey leaf teabag to reduce any swelling. Alternate with ice applications.

Eye Wash   This is a great eye wash. Combine with crushed fennel seed tea and boric acid. Strain. Bathe the eyes.

Wounds   Make up a goldenseal ointment, or combine the dry powder of goldenseal with equal amounts of dry slippery-elm-bark powder; add a minute amount of water, or even spit, to make up into a damp paste. You can also combine goldenseal with plantain ointment or comfrey ointment, depending on the need. All will help in healing and reducing an infection. See the treatment mentioned under Garlic (page 66).

Eruptions   Ringworm, poison ivy, and sudden eruptions respond to continuous washing with or soaking in goldenseal tea.
      Herbal folk medicine also includes the internal use of goldenseal as a bitter tonic to aid internal infection, to cleanse the body after an infection, to aid digestion, to increase bile action, to possibly help clear the body of internal catarrh, and to heal rectal ulcers.

Hawthorn [Crataegus oxycantha]

The hawthorn is a remarkable shrub, and the haws, very much like a miniature apple, can be made into a delicious jelly or simmered to make an excellent diuretic. Hawthorn tonic, available through several reputable pharmacies, has long been thought to be a heart strengthener, to help with weak hearts, fatty heart, or weakness of cardiac muscles. Herbalists throughout the world feel hawthorn helps to reduce edema brought on by heart malfunction. However, you should consult a health professional for heart problems.

Hayflowers/Hayblossoms ★

The blossoms of wild hay of the mountains are an indispensable herbal aid for healing and curative detoxifying baths, ointments, and poultices. I can tell you we regret it when we use up and don't replace our hayflower bath extract (we usually use the great Swiss product put out by BioKosma, and distributed in the United States by Weleda). The hayflowers can be used for foot soaks, hand soaks, or in small amounts in a full bath. A hayflower bath and a vigorous coarse salt rubdown prior to the bath will overcome the fatigue of overwork or overpartying. If you live in the country, make up your own extract. The mixture of mountain hayflowers diluted in water has a profound effect on the skin. In our family experience, hayflower soaks extract toxins, reduce inflammation, help undo party excesses.

Honey (See *My Favorite Herbs.)*

Hops ★

When I was a child we always went to "pine" country during the Christmas holidays, and to this moment I can hear the sleigh bells and the choppity-chop of horses' hooves through the snow. We always brought back aromatic pine pillows. During the rest of the year there were always some hops pillows about the house. A little hops tea and a snooze on a hops pillow will help to get you into a mood for a deep sleep.

Horehound *[Marrubium Vulgare]*

The white horehound is a popular remedy for coughs and

colds and can be used in the form of candy. (See recipes and references to horehound in Section 3.)

Ipecac

Syrup of Ipecac, an ancient folk medicine, is a standard anti-poison substance and should be in every medicine chest. If a child or an adult is poisoned by some substance quickly call your local Poison Control Center (the number should be listed along with your police, fire, ambulance, and physician). They will tell you what substance to use. Having Syrup of Ipecac as an emetic (vomiting agent) may save someone's life.

You can purchase small vials of this syrup in any drugstore. Be sure to keep it out of the easy reach of children.

Jewelweed (See *Poison Ivy.*)

Juniper *[Juniperus communis]* ★

I consider juniper to be one of the most curative of the herb simples. Almost all the parts have some healing power, but I particularly like to use the berries. The berries are gently stimulant and diuretic, and impart to the urine a smell of violets. The berries contain a yellow oil which can act beneficially on the kidneys, and in our family experience is very useful in reducing any tissue swelling. You can obtain about an ounce of the oil from about forty berries.

Juniper is exceptionally cleansing and can be used in combination with most other herbs, except in the case of fever control. To use, crush an ounce of the bruised berries in a pint of boiling water, and drink that tea over the course of twenty-four hours. Or make up a tincture of the berries in vodka or gin (there are juniper berries in gin). Steep for a week or more, then strain out the berries. Use a teaspoonful, well-diluted in water, several times a day. For flatulence, use the juniper berry cure (see page 144). Externally, the tincture can be applied to any painful swellings. Or the bruised berries may be applied in the form of a healing poultice to help relieve neuralgic pains, rheumatic pains, or swellings.

For rheumatism try making up a strong tea of the needles, wood, or bark, and take frequent baths in this juniper. This treatment can be used at any age, and for chronic resistant rheumatism.

Lady's Mantle *(Alchemilla vulgaris)* ★

The word "alchemilla" means magic, and ancient physicians deemed this herb a remarkable and restorative plant for most women's problems. It is very astringent and is good for wounds. In Switzerland the herb has been used to insure sleep, cure headaches, inflammation, toothache (use as a gargle), and as a warm tea to overcome colds of the eyes.

Since the herb is so astringent, it can be used to control excessive and profuse menstrual flow and may also be used along with red raspberry leaf tea for home birth. According to Kunzle, "Every woman in childbed ought to drink a good deal of this herb tea for eight to ten days before giving birth. Many children would still have their mothers, and many a stricken widower his wife, if they had known this gift of God."

Kunzle used this herb tea in large amounts to calm fever and inflammation in the case of any internal injuries. Drink up to two quarts a day. Add honey to accelerate healing.

Lady's Mantle may be mixed with aromatic herbs and used as a beverage tea.

Lavender (English Lavender)
[Lavandula augustifolia formerly *vera]*

Lavender is a lovely aromatic plant that can be purchased in dried form or grown in home gardens. It exudes a resinous camphor, and can be applied hot in compress form to allay local pains. A few drops of the essence of lavender in a hot foot bath will banish fatigue almost immediately! Applied on the body, it will act as a strong stimulant and may relieve various neuralgic pains, sprains, rheumatism, and even the pain of a neuralgic toothache. A few drops of this essence or the lavender oil on the forehead may dispel a headache and conquer minor mental depression. Many households in France keep an essence of lavender to treat painful bruises, bites, and aches.

The most common use of lavender is as an insect repellent. Use it as a fragrant addition to potpourris for closet and drawer sachet. Since mosquitoes and midges hate the smell of lavender, you can deny them access to your person by slipping a cotton ball dipped in lavender into your pocket or by spraying lavender water over the patio.

One of the most refreshing uses of lavender is in a home cosmetic vinegar. Add a handful of lavender flowers to 2 cups of white vinegar or apple cider vinegar. Add 6 cups of rose water. You may add rose petals or jasmine petals. Let the flowers steep for a week, but shake and turn the liquid each day. Strain off the flowers. This vinegar may be used on the face to restore the acid mantle, or on the body to restore energy. Vinegar is an excellent aid for oily skin.

All parts of lavender are fragrant, but oils are made from the flowers. While you don't need a sunny location, and the soil need not be particularly fertile, it must drain well. To dry these flowers pick them before they are completely dry.

Excellent sources of true English lavender (*Lavendula angustifolia* formerly *vera*) can be obtained from plant cuttings from White Flower Farm, Litchfield, Conn., 06759 (mail source), or Martin Viette Nurseries, East Norwich, N.Y.

Licorice *[Glycyrrhiza glabra]*

The root of the licorice plant is used throughout the world mostly to help with chest coughs and to hide the bitter or acrid taste of other medicinal plants.

Ulcers During a recent visit to Japan, I interviewed Dr. Takagi, Dean of Pharmacy, at the University of Tokyo. He was researching the values of ginseng, peony, and licorice. He and his colleagues had concluded that licorice can inhibit gastric secretion, and would be useful for those who had gastric ulcers. Japanese herbalists use the combination of licorice and peony to reduce sharp and intense pain, he told me.

To Release   The root of the plant releases its sweet taste and healing mucilage through boiling in water. The juice can be hardened into different shapes—the origin of the original licorice lozenge.

Tea   To add sweetness, use licorice in any herbal tea. Licorice has the ability to help the system retain fluid. It can be used by thin and dehydrated people to great advantage, but should not be used by those who tend to retain fluid.

Poultice   Simmer licorice sticks and flaxseed together to make a healing paste to use on nonmalignant growths.

Influenza   An old Swiss mountain antiflu remedy: Combine a handful of the bruised licorice root, bruised wormwood leaves, sage leaves, and speedwell to a pint of boiling water. Drink some twice a day during epidemics. Use a spoonful of this preparation every hour if you catch the flu. (Also see Cinnamon and Cayenne in *My Favorite Herbs*.)

Hoarseness and Bronchitis   Simmer sticks of licorice root with such herb teas as peppermint, chamomile, ginger, ginseng, marshmallow, or comfrey. These combinations will gently stimulate the kidneys and bowel function.

Alter Disease State   This is one of the most used herbs in the traditional oriental materia medica. The Chinese feel it normalizes the body (is an alterative) from negative to healthy state.

Hypoglycemia   Some hypoglycemia patients feel relief from symptoms with several cups of licorice tea a day.

Marigold (see Calendula, page 25)

Marjoram (Sweet) *[Origanum marjorana]*

Marjoram tea is a mild tonic, which lessens fever, acts as a stimulant, helps with most digestive problems and is a headache aid. Prepare a poultice by making a hot mash of the leaves, and apply it to sprains, bruises, and for pain.

Swelling and Rheumatism   The ancient Greeks called this plant "joy of the mountains," and used it as an internal and external medicine to relieve painful swellings and rheumatism.

Compress   Marjoram may be used alone or mixed with equal parts of flaxseed and some boiling water. Apply it hot to relieve pain, inflammation, earache and toothache, and for sprains, bruises, and abscesses. To attempt to relieve nervous headache, apply the compress to the head.

Liniment   Combine marjoram, thyme, and olive oil, and use the mixture on sore muscles, charley horse, backache, arthritis, sprain, and bruises.

Sore Throat   To relieve sore throat, dip a cotton cloth into a strong marjoram tea, and wrap the cloth around the throat. Overwrap with a larger, warm flannel cloth. Make it as airtight as possible.

Marshmallows (Mallow, Marsh)
[Althaea officinalis] ★

Marshmallow root (part of the mallow family—mallow means "to soften" in Greek) releases a gummy substance when chewed or simmered in water. This mucilaginous gel is soothing, lubricating, softening, healing, and pain-easing, both internally and externally.

Pain   Apply the softened root to the pain, or add a strained decoction of the root to any foot bath or full bath. To make such a decoction, simmer a quarter of a pound of the dried, cleaned root in two quarts of water, and reduce it to six cups. Strain before using the bath.

Coughs, Hoarseness, and Tonsilitis   The mucilaginous properties of this plant help to alleviate chest congestion. Honey may be added for sweetening.

Stings   Any wild mallow flower is an excellent compress for wasp sting.

Eye Lotion   Prepare an infusion of the leaves and apply it as a compress to reduce inflammation of the eyelid.

Mouth Abscess   Prepare a strong tea of the leaves, and use it as a rinse for an abscess or gum boil.

Mullein (Great) *[Verbascum thapsus]*

As you travel along highways in the United States, tall mullein spikes are visible in wastelands along the roadway. Downy mullein leaves are an age-old folk medicine for chest complaints. Oil from the flowers is often used for ear problems.

Coughs   Gather the leaves in late summer before the plant flowers; tie, hang, and dry the leaves in a cool, airy place. In many parts of Europe and the British Isles, two tablespoons of dried mullein leaves are added to two large cups of milk, simmered for about ten minutes, strained, and drunk warm twice a day to alleviate chest problems. The taste of this preparation is rather gummy, slightly bitter, but restorative.

The dried leaves can also be smoked, or added to other leaves such as coltsfoot or elecampane, to help relieve long-standing coughs, and to help relieve nasal and chest irritations.

Ears   The oil made from the flowers can be purchased from several reliable homeopathic pharmacies and some botanic sources. If you have a stand of mullein, gather the tiny flowers, steep them in olive oil, and stand the oil in the sun for three weeks. Turn the bottle each day.

This preparation is a bactericide. Furthermore, two or three drops of the mullein oil in the ear may alleviate ear pain and help to eliminate dry eczema of the ear. For persistent ear problems, check your health professional.

Bedwetting   My grandmother had a lot of faith in mullein oil to control bedwetting of children. She advised five drops of the oil in a teaspoon of cold water three to four times a day.

Mustard (Black) *[Brassica nigra]*

The dried seeds of the black mustard plant are easily powdered. Dried mustard can be purchased in markets and in drug stores. The powder is one of the most important herbal medicines, in that it will quickly bring blood to the surface of the skin. This rubefacient ability is very useful in preparing poultices to alleviate chest and other congestions, and as an ingredient in hot footbaths to draw chest or nasal congestions or headaches away from the upper extremities. Mustard flour is an antiseptic and a deodorizer for the kitchen.

Foot Bath ★   Add about a tablespoon or more of the dried powder to any hot footbath for a cold in the head, a chest cough, or a headache. The blood will flow away from the overcongested area and rush to the feet. The body soon sends the blood back through normal channels, and proper circulation is restored.

Mustard Poultice (Plaster)   Add one tablespoon of mustard to every four of flour. The more flour, the weaker the plaster or poultice will be. Mix the two ingredients in a bowl and add a very small amount of warm water, just enough to make a nonrunny paste. Fold two large, clean, men's handkerchiefs, or use a dish cloth so that the paste cannot run out. Add the mustard paste, and apply it on the congested chest or painful rheumatic area. Add olive or castor oil to the skin first if the patient has a delicate skin.

These mustard poultices (also called plasters) are invaluable. I have often used them to relieve sudden congestion or rheumatic-type pain. At a party a woman told me of her recent good experience with this poultice. "I worked hard, almost too hard to clear my desk in order to take this planned trip to Turkey, and because of my fatigue came down with a severe laryngitis and extreme tightness of the chest. My physician came over and checked those heavy rumbling chest rales, and knew by the clicking sound he heard through the stethoscope that I had an infection and heavy mucus on my lungs. He told me I could not go on the trip, but he gave me an antibiotic, and agreed to come back to see me in the morning.

"After the doctor left, my husband and I were depressed. After all, we were looking forward to the trip, and it was all paid for in advance. I called my elder sister and cried on the phone, and she said, 'Hey, wait a minute, let's not give up. Maybe mama's remedies could work.' She came over with a box of mustard powder from the drugstore, made it into a poultice, and applied it over my chest and back, all through the night. We kept on shifting it, and honestly, I kept on feeling better and better.

"When the physician came over the next morning, he was stunned to see me up and around, cheerful, and ready for the trip. He said he had never seen antibiotics work so fast. Because I'm prone to chest congestions, I'm never without some mustard powder now."

Myrrh [Commiphora myrrha] ★

Myrrh is a gum resin which exudes from the stem of the myrrh bush. It emerges as a pale yellow liquid, but hardens to a reddish-brown tear no larger than a walnut. The resin has an aromatic smell but a bitter taste; it has excellent astringent and healing properties. While it is solvent in both water and alcohol, the best way to use myrrh is in a tincture form. This tincture is available in drugstores.

Myrrh is marvelous for any mouth problems, and the diluted tincture can be added to water or combined with goldenseal powder to brush the teeth, rinse the mouth, or massage the gums. When combined with goldenseal, it is quite effective on gum problems and mouth sores.

Use diluted myrrh tincture to wash invalids and control the formation of bedsores. Alternate this wash with application of comfrey and/or calendula ointment.

Myrrh is much used in Chinese herbal medicine, especially for wounds and uterine discharges.

Nettle (Stinging nettle) [Urtica urens] ★

The plant is covered by stinging hairs. Each sting causes irritation and inflammation, but—oddly—the juice of the same flowers, as well as other nearby plants such as yellow dock, will instantly cure the sting.

The above-ground part of the herb is a highly praised, cleansing cure-all for the stomach, lungs, and intestines. I know a ninety-five-year-old herbalist who insists that nettle juice or nettle tea will cure ulcers of the stomach and intestines. He combines, and makes a tea of, nettle juice, plantain juice, and juniper berries. He suggests that the tea be sipped warm during the day over a long period of use.

The leaves of the young nettle are delicious in a salad or slightly cooked like young spinach leaves. Nettle has a reputation as a blood cleanser and acts in a tonic fashion.

There is a Father Kneipp nettle juice which can be purchased through gourmet groceries and through some health-food stores and catalogs.

Nutmeg [Myristica fragrans]

I adore the aroma of this herb, and I grate a small amount into many drinks and desserts. My grandmother loved nutmeg tea, and she would often make about a pint of weak tea to inspire sleep. A small amount of fresh grated nutmeg each day has internally warming properties and will help sluggish digestion, flatulence, and diarrhea. Do not use very concentrated or large doses of this aromatic herb, as large amounts of the tea will cause giddiness and intoxication and will produce too deep a sleep. I use fresh grated nutmeg in a wonderful tonic wine (see Section Three).

Steep nutmeg in leftover wine to make an excellent liniment. This is especially good for rheumatic complaints.

Oatmeal *[Avena pativa]* ★

This wonderful food herb is an exceptionally healing poultice-paste for the skin. It may also be blended into finer particles to add to bathwater. Add a small amount of water to make a paste. This paste works on sores, inflammations, and rough skin, and will relieve the itch of hives or poison ivy; it will help soften and draw out splinters and other foreign objects, and will lessen the pain in any infected wound. I have also used the paste to somewhat deaden pain from a swelling, and it can be used to quiet the skin after a chigger or tick is pulled out. "Aveeno" is a prepared pharmaceutical oatmeal which dissolves readily in bathwater. It will take out the sting of hives or itching, and may be used to quiet eczema pain.

Oatmeal porridge is very healing internally and may be used for any invalid or during any convalescence.

Olive *[Olea Europaea]* ★

Olive oil has been used for centuries to help heal lesions within the body, and is used in many parts of the world as a medicine to help expel gallstones. To try to alleviate stomach pains, drink olive oil just before eating to prevent postmeal contractions. Start with a small amount, and work up to a dose of ten to eighteen tablespoons. Chronic stomach pains, of course, should lead you to consult your physician.

Onion [Ailium cepa] ★

For medicinal purposes, onions may be used both internally and externally.

As with garlic and leek, internal use of onion increases circulation and stimulates and warms the body. Use roasted onions as a poultice for earaches, and raw and bruised onions for sprains, bruises, and unbroken chilblains (minor frostbite).

"Where the Lilies Bloom" is a film about orphan children in Appalachia who learn the technique of wildcrofting—picking medicinal herbs for the botanical market. One unforgettable scene shows them saving a neighbor's life by immersing him in a bathtub filled with cut onions. Onions used in this way restore health by forcing intense body "weeping," which releases destructive toxins from the body.

Internal Uses Indian researchers using double-blind controls concluded in *Lancet*, the British medical journal, that onion (and garlic) help to reduce serum cholesterol after a fatty meal. "Both garlic and onion juices have now been found very significant in preventing fat-induced increase in serum cholesterol and plasma fibrinogen. . . . They may prove to be a convenient and safe dietary measure for everyday use in persons who appear to be predisposed to atherosclerosis on account of family history, hyperlipemia, hypertension, or diabetes."

Flu: Note the recipe for onion soup in Section Three. Drink the soup very hot.

Coughs: An old pioneer remedy consists of simmered honey and onion syrup. The onion may be juiced first and added to the honey if this seems more desirable. Add a pinch of thyme and ginseng powder, as both are very helpful in chest complaints.

Aftertaste: To eliminate aftertaste in eating raw onions, Craig Claiborne of *The New York Times* advises:

> After you slice or chop the raw onions, put them in a
> sieve and pour boiling water over them, draining

quickly under cold running water. Or you can put
the prepared onions in a mixing bowl and pour
boiling water over them.

Do this quickly and do not let the pieces steep in the
water. Instead, drain them immediately and add
cold water to cover and a few ice cubes to chill them
quickly. If you do this quickly enough, the onions
will remain crisp and that strong flavor that bothers
will be diminished.

External Uses   Cough: Apply roasted onion to the chest.
    Sinus: Inhale fresh cut onion until the nasal passages are
unclogged.
    Bruises: Hold a fresh cut onion to the bump, bruise, or
ankle or elbow sprain, and the pain will be relieved. For large
areas, place the cut onion on the body, cover the area with a
sheet of plastic wrap, and attach it to the body with a large
elastic bandage. To increase the effect of the onion on sprains,
combine equal parts of onion and common salt.
    Hemorrhoids: Another old English remedy is the use of
raw, bruised onions. Attach a portion to protruding or inflamed hemorrhoids for relief of pain.
    Chilblains: Combine salt and raw onions. Pound them
together, and apply the result to unbroken skin. For skin
showing lesions, use *no* salt and apply roasted onions.

Papaya

Stings   Use papaya enzyme or Adolph's Meat Tenderizer,
which contains papaya, to relieve the pain and inflammation
of a wasp or hornet sting.

Infection   Strips of fresh papaya pulp may be used over
weeping sores of any kind. The enzyme in the papaya clears
up the pus in a short while.

Digestion ★   Papaya enzymes are an excellent digestive aid. Purchase fresh papaya juice or papaya tablets.

Parsley *[Carum petroselinum]*

Diuretic ★   Parsley may be eaten raw, juiced in an extractor, or made into a soup to produce a free flow of urine from the system.

Poultice   To soften hard breasts in the early stage of nursing, apply bruised parsley to the breasts.

Peaches

Internal Use   Peach pit, peach twig, and peach flower tea produce a volatile oil somewhat similar to the poisonous bitter almond. These substances are sometimes used by knowledge-able herbalists, but I would advise the novice to avoid internal use. The flower tea is purgative.

External Uses   During the peach season make peach pit tea and keep it in the refrigerator (label: External). It is very healing, cleansing, and will often allay the pain of wounds. The pits can be cooked and added to alcohol or glycerine to preserve the juice. *Be sure to mark "for external use only."*

Worms   One surprising use of peach leaves is as a poultice to help extract worms from children. Add a small amount of boiling water to the leaves, just enough to release its chemicals and make it into a paste. Apply the mash to the child's stomach. Cover the area with plastic wrap and a large towel. Use for half-hour intervals once a day for as long as needed.

Pennyroyal *[Mentha Pulegium]*

Pennyroyal oil is a strong insect repellent and is often

used by herbalists as such on leather soaked dog collars. It can be strong and irritating for sensitive skin however.

A word of *caution* on the use of pennyroyal oil for any *internal* use—some misinformed herbal advisers have suggested its use as an abortifacient, and it has been used in Colorado for this purpose. Several fatal accidents have occurred as a result of its use. *Do NOT use it internally!*

Peppermint (See *My Favorite Herbs.*)

Pine ★

Pine needle extract is readily available in drug departments. Even in small quantities, it is a remarkable addition to a bath, for it helps to alleviate pain and joint discomfort and overcomes the feeling of fatigue. The aroma itself is stimulating and calming.

Many folk remedies contain turpentine, the virgin resin that drips out of scarred white pine. This herbal terpentine is not to be confused with the common "boiled" turpentine available through hardware stores, which is *not* for use in herbal medicine.

Plantain (Common) *[Plantago major]*

Even if you live in a city, you can find this weed in any local park or wayside. The Greek physician Dioscorides in the 1st century A.D. describes how this green plant was used externally by the Roman army on body sores. A neighbor of mine once developed a terrible finger infection from a manicure "nick." Despite emergency-room lancing and constant use of antibiotics, it wouldn't heal. We walked to a nearby park, picked up some plantain, and wrapped her throbbing finger. She felt almost immediate relief. We took home a batch of this low-growing weed and placed the leaves in water, so she would have a constant renewable bandage for this infection. Using it, the infection cleared in a few days.

Apply the leaves to the face to relieve some earaches, or chew it, gargle with it, or drink plantain tea for relief of a toothache.

Use the leaves to relieve the pain of bee, wasp, and hornet stings.

Potato

Burn, Bruise, Sprain   I hope you keep raw potatoes around your house, because they can be very helpful in first aid. Use a raw, peeled, grated potato around an eye bruise or a sprain of any kind, and sometimes to relieve the pain of a minor burn. An old-fashioned Viennese physician tells me he prescribes the application of the hot baked potato pulp for tennis elbow or any other joint pain.

Potatoes are alkaline within the body, and, like string beans, parsley, zucchini, squash, and celery, should be part of an alkaline-detoxifying diet. Carrots are also alkaline, but should be used separately. ★

Raspberry (See *My Favorite Herbs.*)

Rose Hips ★

Rose hips have several medicinal uses in addition to being high in vitamin C. Try to make rose hip tea a part of your daily diet.

The woolly down enveloping the hips can sometimes shove round worms from the system. Father Kunzle, the Swiss herbalist, also recommends the use of rose hips to help expel kidney stones.

Rosewater

I make up my own rosewater with a small amount of rose oil and distilled water. This is useful added to apple cider vinegar to make up cosmetic vinegar, for eye washes, for my favorite homemade cold cream, and as a delicate yet non-allergic aroma for some ointments. Rosewater is available from pharmacists, botanical sources, and Mideast food shops.

Sage (Common) *[Salvia officinalis]*

"We are happier in many ages when we are old, than when we are young. The young sow wild oats, the old grow sage!" (Winston Churchill). That's a lovely play on words, and I hope we all do grow sage, for it is an amazing herb and is one of the greatest tonics and curative herbs. It is useful for health purposes, including sleep, gargles, breath cleansing, fever, rough skin, sprains, as a mild diuretic, as part of an anti-infection vinegar wash, to cleanse the smell of a sickroom, to help heal leg ulcers, as an antiseptic, and as a tea to lift mild depression. No wonder it means "to save," in Latin. It is one of my panacea herbs.

Depression Drink sage tea to lift a down mood. If available, add a pinch of bruised cloves and a pinch of pure ginseng powder (another antidepression herb).

Breath Rub the sage leaves across the teeth to cleanse them and give a sweet smell to the breath, as many Arabs, American Indians, and Far Eastern Indians do.

Fever The American Indians used sage tea rubdowns and sage baths, and this antifever remedy seems to exist all over the world. I sometimes like to combine apple cider vinegar and sage tea for reduction of fever and to make the patient simply feel better.

Give the patient lots of sage tea to drink. Lemon juice and honey may be added in small amounts if desired. Hot sage tea will produce slight perspiration, and this is useful in helping to reduce fever. Make sure to sponge the body with cold water friction sectional rubs that allow only one part of the body to be exposed at a time.

Antiseptic ★   Chew sage leaves to cleanse the system of impurities. Prepare a strong sage tea to cleanse the sickroom—this is quite helpful when children are ill. Sage is one of the antiseptic herbs in the Vinegar of the Four Thieves.

Gargle   Add a few sage leaves to plain water, or add five sage leaves to a glass of leftover white or red wine. Several longer-lasting sage and other herbal gargles are mentioned in other parts of this book.

Sleep   Sage was always part of my grandmother's "sleep" jar. She combined several aromatic and sleep-inducing herbs, including peppermint, chamomile, skullcap, bruised cloves, rose hips, and linden.

Stomach Troubles   Use cold sage tea.

Flu   Kunzle used sage, wormwood, licorice root, and alpine speedwell (a handful of each) in his famous antiflu remedy. He suggests its use before and during epidemics and to hasten healing during a flu attack.

Pleurisy   Combine a handful of sage leaves and corn silk to strengthen the kidneys and expel water from the system. If you like, you may add a pinch of rue leaves to quicken the blood circulation.

Varicose Veins, Ulcers on the Legs   Apply hot sage compresses, use sage washes on the leg, and take frequent sage footbaths.

Senna *[Cassia acutifolia]*

Senna is a strong herbal purgative. I recently read a report from the Center for Disease Control noting its misuse by a family who thought it was just "another" herbal tea. They gave it to a child, with disastrous results. BEFORE YOU

DRINK ANY BLEND OF HERBS, FIND OUT WHAT THE
BLEND IS DESIGNED FOR. IF YOU CAN'T FIND OUT, AND
YOU DON'T KNOW ALL THE HERBS, DON'T DRINK THE
BLEND!

Incidentally, if you need a herbal laxative, Innerclean and
Swiss Kriss are both mild and effective.

Shepherd's Purse *[Capsella bursa-pastoris]*

This insignificant little weed may be a lifesaver to you and
your friends some day, as it is an excellent styptic. It will stop
bleeding when some ordinary remedies don't work. Bruise the
plant and apply it on the wound. Or prepare the whole plant
as a tea, drink it, and apply it as a wash to the wound.

Slippery Elm (Bark) *[Ulmus fulva]*

Powdered slippery elm lozenges are available for sore
throats, and they are quite healing. The powder made from the
inner bark can also be purchased from botanical sources. This
is an exceptionally healing substance. It can be used as a paste
and applied to sores, bruises, wounds, or mixed with other
healing herbs in ointment or paste. I like it mixed with comfrey
root ointment or calendula lotion or ointment, and I sometimes
mix it with goldenseal, as a paste. Kloss, in *Back to Eden*, is
strong in his praise of this herb and suggests its use as a
suppository for vaginal problems.

Strawberry (See *My Favorite Herbs.*)

Thyme (See *My Favorite Herbs.*)

Valerian *(Valeriana officinalis)*

This is an interesting plant. The root has the medicinal
value, and it can be used as a tea, as a poultice, or in pill form.

The most important use of valerian is as a tranquilizer, and it was used for this purpose during the Blitz in England during World War II. Valerian may be used to try to overcome body spasms, to sedate an anxious or overstressed person, or to overcome a crying spell.

Culpeper added valerian root to raisins, aniseeds, and licorice for a cough quieter, and other herbalists use the tincture of valerian, or a poultice from the roots, for compress relief on painful rheumatic or swollen joints. It may also be used in bathwater for this same purpose.

While the root doesn't smell wonderfully to us, it is powerfully attractive to cats and rats. Some think the legendary Pied Piper of Hamelin may have carried valerian root hidden on his body.

I like valerian in a tiny discote (pill), and thus far I think the best of these pills come from Kiehl's Pharmacy, Third Avenue and 13th Street, New York City. "Bio-Nutritional Products", P.O. Box 389, Harrison, New York, 10528, sells the organic Walther Schoenberger (fresh) valerian juice.

Tincture of Valerian To make your own tincture for bath or compress:

> 4 ounces of the valerian powder
> 2 pints ninety-proof alcohol
> additional for dilution

Moisten the fine powder, dilute it slightly with the additional alcohol. Pack the powder into a Chemex "coffee" parchment and pour the 2 pints of ninety-proof alcohol over the herb. Let it drip down. Strain out any powder that has seeped through, and pass the alcohol through the powder once again. Pour the liquid into a dark, labeled jar.

Compress Dilute some tincture, heat it up, and pour over a folded cloth, and apply somewhat dry, but hot, to swollen joints.

Bath   Add some drops of tincture to a warm bath to relieve pain of rheumatic attack.

Witch Hazel *(Hamamelis virginiana)*

Americans learned how to use this extraordinary herb from the Indians who made a decoction (from the twigs) for swellings, inflammations, and tumors. Today millions of gallons of this extract are sold around the world. It is a good item to keep in the medicine chest as it will instantly reduce swelling from swollen or tired eyes, relieve the pain of sunburn—and can be used as a shave lotion. It can be used in a douche to check excessive white discharges or menstrual flow. Use it as a face splash for oily skin and to control minor pimple formation.

Witch hazel will quickly reduce the pain from any insect bite and should be used cold, along with ice, to reduce the pain of sprains or athletic injuries. It is even used in some hospital recovery rooms to reduce swelling from intravenous feeding.

Wormwood *[Artemisia Absinthium]*

This is a potent herb. Use a tiny sprig or some dried leaves in various teas, or in tonic wines as a digestive aid. (It is also used in the bitter apertif Campari.) Apply diluted wormwood tincture, or strong wormwood tea, in a compress to heal bruises and ease the pain of a fall or an accident of any kind. (See Resource list for fresh wormwood herbal juice.)

Yarrow *(Achillea millefolium)*

This is an old wound herb and was supposed to be a favorite herb of Achilles. It is a great insect repellent; use it splashed over the body in the tea form, or rub the flowers on the body to repel mosquitoes while you are in the country.

Since it is a very common weed, it will be easy to recognize, so get to know it.

I use small amounts of the flowers, or the fresh (German) Juice in my anticold, perspiration-inducing teas with ginger, peppermint, elderflower, and ginseng. It also helps to cleanse the liver.

Yarrow tea makes a good mouthwash for canker sores. It is said to tighten the uterus and to cause contractions to bring down the afterbirth during childbirth, so it is contra-indicated for pregnant women, as far as I am concerned.

Important

Please refer to the Special Notice to the Reader on page xx and the instructions on page 117.

SECTION TWO

A HERBAL SELECTOR

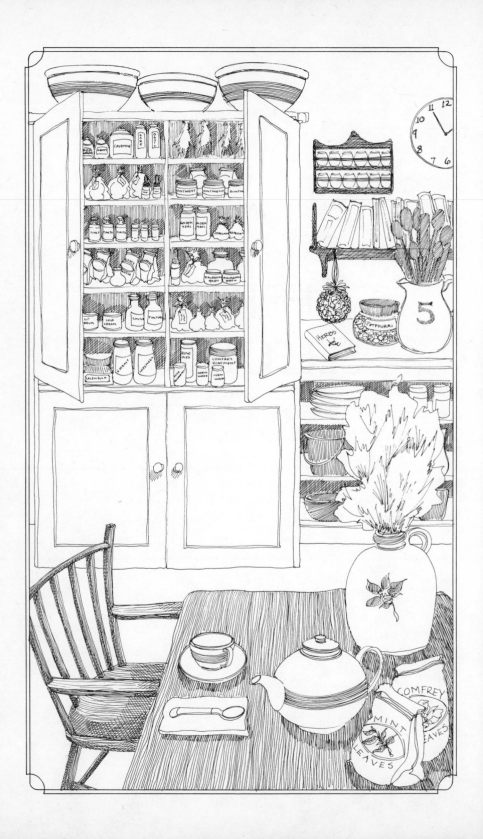

While the ailments listed below may not necessarily be cured by the herbal treatments given, they may at least be alleviated. Any serious or chronic conditions should of course be reported to your physician or health professional and he or she should be consulted lest any herbal treatment here be counter to a course of treatment he or she has prescribed.

In ministering to infants, first test moderate amounts of a herbal remedy cautiously. Do not feed uncooked honey to infants under one year of age.

Important

Please refer to the Special Notice to the Reader on page xx and the instructions on page 117.

ALCOHOL ABUSE

Angelica A decoction of the root, or several grains of the powdered root, is an old folk remedy for developing a disgust for liquor.

Cayenne ★ To wean away from liquor, combine a few drops of tincture of cayenne (tincture of capsicum) and a few drops of tincture of orange peel and water. A few grains of the pepper may be added to hot herbal drinks for restorative and stimulative action.

Chamomile Chamomile tea is said to help offset some reactions to alcohol drinking.

Watercress ★ Counteract postparty fatigue and alcoholic fumes by eating lots of watercress. Watercress is also useful to offset the smell and taste of smoking. The pure, pressed juice of watercress is imported from Germany.

ALLERGIES

Use comb honey and eat honey in three-day cycles several weeks before hay fever attacks are expected to occur. When possible, utilize honey made in the area in which you live. Honey and apple cider vinegar (1 tablespoon of each) diluted in a full glass of water is an excellent, restorative, and balancing drink. ★

Ginseng   Small amounts of ginseng powder added to herbal drinks may help overcome the propensity for allergic attacks, especially hayfever or sinus.

ANEMIA

Each day drink ¼ cup of beet juice added to some fresh carrot juice.

ANTISEPTICS

Thousands of plants have antiseptic value, and many have active antibiotic ingredients. For home and outdoors, use the following herbs and recipes.

Cabbage   White cabbage leaves contain rapine, an antibiotic active against some fungi. White cabbage leaves have an affinity for pus or ulcers to absorb pus. Break down the large thread veins, warm the leaves, and place them on the sore. Replace when warm.

Carrot   Boil carrots, mash them, and apply them to sores to extract pus and heal the area. Carrots are a very strong antiseptic.

Cinnamon Bark   Cinnamon bark contains an active fragrant, volatile, antigermicidal oil. Use the bark in mouthwashes, gargles, combinations of herbal teas for taste and antiseptic ability.

Clove   Clove oil, like cinnamon bark oil, is a strong germicide; both are considered more powerful than carbolic acid. Use bruised cloves in teas and externally to deaden skin pain.

(Sweet) Clover   These attractive wayside weeds contain a broad spectrum antibiotic.

Creosote (Bush)   This plant contains nordihydroguaiaretic acid, an antibiotic active against skin bacteria.

(Red) Currant   Heat the juice of the red currant over a slow fire for an old-fashioned dessert, "Rob," or as the ancient English remedy for sore throat. Red currant jelly may be added to peppermint or ginger tea as an anti-sore throat aid.

Garlic   Extracts of garlic buds contain allicin, a powerful antibacterial agent. In Russia during World War II, in the absence of penicillin and other antibiotics, the Russians used garlic powder on wounds. For a tasty anticold remedy, combine finely cut beefsteak tomatoes, red onions, mashed garlic buds, vegetable oil, and lemon juice. Eat as much as you can stand. (See "Garlic" and "Onions" for additional details.)

Ginger   Wild ginger contains a broad-spectrum antibiotic active against bacteria and fungi. Ginger root or ginger powder added to herbal drinks at the onset of a cold causes perspiration and alleviates cold symptoms. Do not use in great amounts. Use a small amount in bathwater, too.

Goldenseal   The root of goldenseal contains berberine, an antibiotic with broad-spectrum antibacteria and antiprotozoa activity. Goldenseal is especially useful for mouth and gum problems. Use the powder of the root directly on canker sores, or combine it with tincture of myrrh and water or sherry for a healing mouthwash.

Horseradish   There is an active antibiotic in the horseradish root. Note the various apple cider vinegar and horseradish recipes and drinks, particularly for sinus problems, in Section Three.

Juniper   The berries have many uses in home herbal care. They contain an antibiotic.

Onions   Onions have always been known to have antibacterial action. Since cut onions easily absorb bacteria, they can be used in a sickroom for this purpose. However, note that this also means that in average home use cut onions should always be completely covered and kept in the refrigerator. See also anticold salad (Garlic) above. Onion broth is restorative. Roasted onion may be used as an effective poultice. To reduce the aftertaste of raw onions, note recipe under internal use *Onions*.

Radish   One old English folk remedy for boils utilized placement of a slice of radish on the boil. Do not eat wild radish seeds.

Sage   Add sage leaves to tea or gargles for sore throat and other antiseptic action. Steep 2 tablespoons in a pint of boiling water for seven to ten minutes. Sage may be bitter if allowed to steep too long in boiling water. (See *sage gargles* in Section Three.)

Thyme   The oil extracted from fresh thyme is complex and contains thymol, which is an exceptionally antiseptic substance similar in antiseptic action to carbolic acid. Thymol may be used in miniscule amounts (one part to a thousand of water) for the dressing of wounds. It is successful even when iodine or other such antiseptics have proved unsuccessful. Though not as potent as the oil, garden thyme can be crushed, added to boiling water, steeped, then strained, and used for baths, compresses, and directly on the body for sprains and bruises.

ARTHRITIS

Take apple cider vinegar baths. Or take ginger root baths. Drink a small amount of ginger tea while in the bath. Drink burdock root, or burdock burr tea: 1 cup three times a day, for a month and a half. Alternate with other cleansing teas, and use detoxification procedures. Arthritis is a systemic problem; consult a health professional versed in the holistic approach to medicine. ★

ASTRINGENT HERBS

Astringents check excessive internal or external secretions, and can tighten and contract the skin and mucus membranes. Astringents may be used for gargles, washes, lotions, mouthwashes, douches, enemas, teas, ointments, and suppositories. The most active astringent herbs are oak bark, bayberry bark, red raspberry, white poplar, witch hazel, yellow dock, cranesbill or wild alum, or wild geranium. For hemorrhoids these high-tannin herbs can be prepared as an ointment and a suppository. Add it to gargles, or make it into a sore throat paint with the addition of glycerine. Add it to mouth washes or toothpastes to overcome mouth infections or pyorrhea.

BEDWETTING

Marjoram   Wild marjoram tea is said to help bedwetting problems as well as nightmares.

Mullein   Use 5 drops of this flower oil (available from certain pharmacies) in a teaspoon of cold water. Stir. Use a teaspoon four times a day for nighttime bedwetting.

St. John's Wort   Also called hypericum: Prepare a tea with an ounce of the flowers to a pint of boiling water to try to overcome nighttime bedwetting. The herb is also an exceptional first aid for wounds, bleeding, and bruises. The flowers give off a red juice. The oil can be obtained by suspending a tightly closed glass jar of the flowers in the sun.

BITES

Treat stings and bites immediately. Withdraw the sting and press out the poison. Wash the wound with cold water if available. Apply wet clay poultice to relieve pain if you are outdoors. Use a lighted match to help knock off ticks.

Banana   Apply banana and oatmeal pack after chigger heads and body are flicked from the victim's body. Note: Chiggers drown in castor oil.

Castor Oil   See above.

Clay   Make a clay paste with clay and water or damp earth and water, and apply it to the areas of bite or sting to relieve the pain.

Feverfew   Make a finely blended powder of this wayside weed that looks like clumps of miniature daisies. Apply the powder to the face and body to keep away mosquitoes and flies. To make a lotion: Make up a tincture of 2 teaspoons of the plant in brandy. Steep for fourteen days. Add drops of the tincture to cold water, and sponge the water over the body.

Garlic   Use a garlic or onion slice on ant bite to balance the acid. Apply cucumber juice afterward to further soothe the pain.

Marigold   Use pot marigold (calendula) petals on bee sting.

Oatmeal   Use oatmeal, or oatmeal and banana paste on the victim's body after chiggers and ticks have been knocked off.

Onion   A slice of onion will immediately relieve the pain of a bee sting.

Plantain   When outdoors, take out the bee or hornet sting, press out the poison, add salad oil if possible, and cover the area with wet, rinsed plantain leaf. Replace the leaf as it dries.

Rue   Apply ice to a snake bite. Place the rue leaves in beer. Drink a little, and also apply the beer to the bite. Rush the victim to a hospital. This is a possible allergenic substance.

Wormwood, Rue, Sage   Apply pulped leaves of either wormwood, sage, or rue, or soak a compress in oils of wormwood, rue, or sage, to alleviate pain of spider, scorpion, or jellyfish bites. Note: This is an important medicine-chest item in high spider, scorpion or jellyfish areas. Some allergic people may be sensitive to wormwood or rue.

BLEEDING AND CUTS

Cayenne Pepper   Cayenne pepper has surprising and immediate internal and external styptic action. A tiny bit of the powder can stop bleeding from a cut, and a really small amount (⅛ of a teaspoon in a large glass of water) has been known to have a profound effect on internal bleeding.

Juniper Berries   While outdoors, pack mashed green juniper berries on a bleeding wound.

Lemon   Although lemon juice will sting, it has an immediate styptic effect, even when ice and other herbs have failed. Midwives once used diluted lemon juice to stem uterine hemorrhage after delivery.

Marigold   *Calendula officinalis* flowers are very useful in all bleeding conditions. Use a few drops of the tincture in clear, cool, boiled water, and wash the wound. The expressed juice may be safely used directly on the wound. Keep the perishable fresh juice of the flowers *(Succus calendula)* in your refrigerator.

Puff Ball   One mushroom, the *Lycoperdon giganteum bovista*, is a successful styptic. When the mushroom is ripe, rub it into a fine powder to stop bleeding of slight wounds and cuts; for larger wounds, bind the puff ball over the wound and leave it until healing takes place. Up to the early part of this century, English villagers kept dried puff ball pieces for wound emergencies.

Red Raspberry   Drink red raspberry leaf tea during pregnancy and during delivery.

Sanicle   "He who has sanicle, or prunella, or bugle plants need have no dealings with a doctor," notes an old English saying. Use any of these bruised wild plants for wound poultice while outdoors. To make up the poultice in advance, steep *Prunella vulgaris* in wine, or collect the expressed juice in small jars, and seal the container with paraffin. Use bugle as a tea, an ointment, or use it crushed and wet as a poultice.

Shepherd's Purse   Even city dwellers can find this common weed in parks. (Plantain is another commonly found weed.) This plant has been used for centuries as an exceptional styptic. Make a tea of the whole plant (a handful to a pint of water) for drinking purposes; use it directly on the wound as a poultice, or add it to bathwater if this is feasible.

BLISTERS

Apply peach pit tea to the blister. Ice applications are also very effective.

BOILS AND ABSCESSES

Cabbage   Break large ridges. Dip the leaves in warm water. Apply. Replace when warm.

Fig   Split fig and apply hot. This is especially effective for a boil on the gum.

Honey   Honey is a strong antibiotic and has been used from earliest times for wounds and boils. Mix honey with a tiny amount of flour, and apply it to bring a boil to a head.

Onion   The Cheyenne Indians used a poultice of onion bulbs and stems. When the boil came to a head, they washed out the pus with raw onion juice and water.

Peach   Make up a strong tea by steeping two peach pits in a cup of boiling water; simmer for ten minutes. Apply the tea as a compress to the boil. Also drink the tea for cleansing action. Make up a peach pit tincture during peach season. Use a few drops diluted in water for tea or compress.

Radish   Many European countries used sliced root of radish on large boils.

Slippery Elm   The powdered fawn-colored bark of this tree is very healing as a poultice, and was widely used by many North American Indian tribes for wounds, boils, and skin diseases. Add cold or tepid water to the powder in small amounts to make a paste.

Thyme   Heat up a strong thyme tea (one handful of thyme to a pint of boiling water). Steep. Dip in a folded cloth. Apply the thyme compress to the abscess, boil, or swellings. Repeat as often as necessary.

BREASTS

Breast Infection   Apply continuous packs of strong peach tea.

Hard Breasts   Apply bruised parsley leaves as a poultice. This is helpful during early lactation.

Caked Breasts   Apply strong peppermint tea compresses.

BRUISES

Agrimony   Crushed roots and leaves may be used on bruises. A French water, Eau de Arquebusabe, made of agrimony, was once used on wounds from early handguns *(arquebuses)*. Agrimony tea may be used for sprains and bruises.

Arnica   The *Arnica montana* is a remarkable bruise remedy. I always keep an arnica tincture, lotion, and ointment on hand for emergency, and I find it very effective on bruises where the skin is unbroken (sprains, blows). Arnica may be used in foot or arm baths, for compress water, or directly on the skin.

Cabbage   Break the ridges on the large outer leaves of white cabbage. Dip the leaves into very hot water, and apply them to bring down face swelling, or to withdraw pus from running sores.

Caraway   Bruise the seeds, heat them with hot, soft bread, and apply this to black and blue marks.

Comfrey   This is one of the most important of the antibruise plants, as it is *exceptionally* healing in every one of its forms. Apply it in compress or poultice form on the bruise. A few drops of the tincture in water can be used to soak inflamed or painful bruises.

Daisy The lovely and common daisy was once called bruisewort. To reduce swelling, bruise the leaves and flowers, and add them to wheat germ oil, or use them as tea.

Mullein The oil made from the flowers of mullein and olive oil is useful for bruises, frostbite, and hemorrhoids.

Onion Onions have exceptional drawing power and may be used in raw or roasted form to help heal bruises.

Shepherd's Purse Use the whole plant as a poultice for painful bruises. (This plant is also useful for rheumatism, and helps to stop bleeding.)

Solomon's Seal Use the crushed root as a poultice to take away black and blue marks on a wound and to help with bruises about the eye. If beer is available, steep the root in the beer, and apply this compress to bruise.

Vinegar Poultice Apply an apple cider vinegar compress to bruises, swelling, or sprains. It may be used hot or cold. Do *not* use this near the eyes or genitals.

Witch Hazel American Indians used twigs of the witch hazel tree to make up tea to reduce swelling and tumors. Distilled witch hazel is available in every drugstore, and compresses dipped in the preparation will quickly relieve minor burns, swellings, and inflammations.

Yarrow This common weed has been used for centuries crushed on fresh cuts and bruises or, added to a lard ointment, to heal bruises.

BURNS

Aloe Vera   This easy-to-grow, succulent houseplant contains a marvelous healing gel within its fleshy leaves. Open the leaf, put it on the burn, sore, or chapped area.

Blueberry   Prepare an extract of blueberry or huckleberry during the season, and use it for burn emergencies, scalds, and eczema lesions.

Potato   Peel and cut raw potatoes, and place them on the burn or scald.

Water   Burns dehydrate the body quickly. If it is only a minor burn, give the burn victim drinking water. Add a pinch of cayenne pepper to the water to help against the shock. Ice water compress or application is very effective for most minor burns.

CHAPPED HANDS

Leek   Blend the juice of a fresh leek into your favorite cream, and use it to overcome chapped hands.

Oatmeal   Uncooked oatmeal blended into fine particles, or cooked oatmeal, or the suspended particles of oatmeal (colloidal oatmeal, Aveeno brand) can be made into a thin paste to soften and heal chapped hands. Add it to bathwater, also. Oatmeal heals many skin eruptions.

Aloe vera ★   Apply the gel from the inside of the leaves of this houseplant to heal chapped hands, skin lesions, or minor burns.

CHILBLAIN (MINOR FROSTBITE)

Cayenne ★   Avoid frostbite or the effect of cold by adding cayenne pepper and an inert powder, such as cornstarch or talcum powder, to the inside of shoes or ice skates. Cayenne keeps the body warm. Add a pinch of cayenne to hot herbal drinks before going outdoors.

Ginger   Drink weak ginger tea, bathe in weak ginger baths, and add ginger powder to shoes (as above) to avoid feeling cold.

Onion   Roast an onion for a poultice on minor frostbite, broken skin, and chilblains. If the skin istill unbroken, you may use a raw onion on the skin.

Potato   Add a small amount of vegetable oil to the inside "meat" of a baked white potato, and apply the potato to the frostbite area.

Prevention: Water ★   Bathe the feet and hands frequently in really cold water to develop a resistance to the cold.

Miscellaneous   Wear layers of clothing and a hat during extremely cold weather. Do *not* drink alcoholic substances.

COLDS

Combine water therapy, such as full hot baths and mustard foot baths, with the following herbs and herb teas to induce perspiration and eliminate body toxins. If a cold persists, a health professional had best be consulted.

Anise   For Infants: Bruise 2 ounces of anise seeds in a mortar, place them in a pitcher, and pour 2 cups of boiling water over the seeds. Steep this for fifteen minutes, cool, and strain. Feed the liquid to the infant in teaspoon doses. Use 1 teaspoon for a one-year-old, up to 3 teaspoons for children over four years of age.

Balm   Fresh balm (melissa) tea will induce perspiration and reduce mild fever. Only use fresh balm, as the dried herb has only minor value.

Barley Water   Wash 2 ounces of barley and discard the water. Boil this barley in 1 pint of water for brief time. Discard the water once again. Place the barley in 4 pints of water and add washed lemon peel: boil the contents down to 2 pints. Strain this and add 2 ounces of honey. Use this freely, especially for children and feeble invalids.

Borage   This plant, much used in France, has high amounts of potassium, calcium, and other minerals, which gives it a refreshing quality. Borage tea stimulates the kidneys, and this is most useful in feverish conditions. Borage is also a refrigerant—it cools the body.

Cayenne Pepper (Also for Flu) ★   Cayenne is one of the extraordinary panacea herbs. It can establish a harmonious balance within the body. When used in small or larger amounts along with other anticold herbs, such as peppermint, balm, yarrow, elderblossoms, or (the bitter) boneset, it will bring on needed perspiration, which will eliminate body poisons and bacteria. Note the excellent cayenne antiflu remedy in the *My Favorite Medical Herbs* section.

Cinnamon   Note the antiflu remedy in the *My Favorite Medical Herbs* section.

Garlic ★   I add several mashed garlic buds to salads, especially a finely cut tomato and red onion salad (with lemon and safflower oil) to help overcome the feeling of an oncoming cold. If the cold produces fever and you vomit, cleanse the intestinal tract and reduce the fever with a garlic enema, made by mashing and blending two garlic buds into some water and adding that to a pint of water.

Ginseng   Add ⅛ teaspoon or a pinch of pure ginseng powder to any of the anticold herbal teas. Ginseng is an herbal alternative which means it will help restore the glands and the rest of the body to a normal, healthy, more energetic state. It is also useful for bad coughs.

Honey   Add honey to hot lemonade for a cough or a cold. Or use a dollop of honey in any of the relevant herbal teas. Honey is a bactericide, an agent that destroys bacteria.

Lemon ★   Lemon is one of the most effective medicines and body cleansers. Wash and cut lemons. Squeeze them into a large pitcher. Add washed halves. Add lots of boiling water. Steep. (Hot lemonade.)
        Add honey to taste, or drink the mix in its sour state. Lemonade is refreshing and restorative. Honey-lemon water is also useful for bad coughs.

Peppermint ★   Peppermint added to other teas adds a marvelous minty and aromatic flavor; it helps settle and cleanse the stomach, reduce spasms, and, in the right combination (½ peppermint, pinches of yarrow, elderblossom, etc.), will help bring on needed perspiration. Use it in bed, after a hot bath, to help eliminate cold symptoms.

Mustard   Mustard powder from mustard seeds can be made into a paste with flour and warm water and applied in a cloth (as a poultice-plaster) to bring blood to the surface of the skin. Mustard powder may be added to foot baths to help decongest the nasal passages.

Yarrow   I often use the pressed fruit juice or dried flowers of this common weed, combined with other herbs, to induce perspiration and eliminate cold symptoms.

CONSTIPATION

Apple Apples contain a great many nutritious and needed minerals. Apples are easily digested and are quite effective in a mono- (one food only) fast to cleanse the body.

Clove Do *not* use cloves in herbal teas if the patient is prone to constipation.

Figs ★ Eat raw or dry figs, as the seeds of the fig help push waste materials through the system, and also act as a laxative.

Honey ★ Honey is not only nutritious, but slightly laxative.

Licorice ★ Add sticks of licorice to any herbal tea for a slight laxative action.

Prunes ★ Prunes and prune juice are laxative.

Spinach ★ Raw spinach salads add needed vitamins and minerals to a diet, and act in a slightly laxative fashion.

Strawberry Strawberries are slightly laxative. Strawberry leaves, however, are useful in controlling extreme diarrhea.

COUGHS–BRONCHITIS–ASTHMA

With proper herbal (and water therapy) treatment, most chest involvements should not go beyond the early stage. Strengthen the total body with daily cold foot-splashes or treading. Add seeds of anise, cloves, nutmeg, and licorice sticks to herbal drinks on a preventive level. Use any of the following herbs, depending on the respiratory condition: ★

Almond Drink Grind several almonds into powder, and

steep that in a pint of cold water. This is a nutritious drink for fever and will help "soften" the cough.

Anise   Make an anise tincture by crushing a handful of anise seeds in a pint of inexpensive brandy. Steep this for two weeks, then strain out the seeds. Use a teaspoon of the resulting liquid at a time added to hot water or hot herbal drink (peppermint, for instance). An excellent (but more complex) tincture of anise is available as anisette liqueur. Purchase a bottle in the liquor store, and keep it on hand for emergencies. Use several tablespoons of anisette, and dilute it with a small amount of water to soothe the hacking of chronic bronchitis or to help alleviate an asthmatic attack. This is usually very effective.

Benzoin (Tincture)   The tears of this resinous tree are an excellent aid for coughs. Buy it in tincture form in a drugstore, and add it to the vaporizer "well." The fumes help alleviate minor chest conditions and also help to clear the skin of impurities.

Camphorated Oil   Purchase oil of camphor in the drugstore, and rub it on the chest to bring blood to the surface and ease chest pain.

(Wild) Cherry   Add a teaspoon of wild cherry bark extract to any herbal drink, such as chamomile, linden (lime blossoms), peppermint, horehound, and so on. It will relieve an irritable cough. The extract is available in health-food stores, gourmet sections of food stores, and some drugstores.

Coltsfoot   Coltsfoot, once such a famous herbal simple that it was the symbol for all apothecaries in France, is now practically unknown. Yet this common weed can also be grown in the garden. Make a tea of the leaves with licorice and honey to alleviate coughs. Coltsfoot leaves may be smoked like tobacco to cure a cough. A well-known British herbal tobacco contains half coltsfoot leaves and small amounts of dried leaves and flowers of the herbs eyebright, thyme, lavender, chamomile, buckthorn, and betony. It is smoked in various parts of Europe to alleviate asthma attacks.

Another coltsfoot cough tea includes a half ounce each of coltsfoot leaves, horehound leaves, comfrey root, hyssop, and vervain, with one stick of licorice. Steep the mixture in 3 pints of boiling water, and stand it for half a day. Use this tea in teaspoon doses throughout the day.

Dock (Yellow Curled)   A few drops of yellow curled dock tincture in a hot herbal tea will help with a tickling cough.

Elecampane   The root of this stunning yellow flower is the basis of many ancient cough medicines and sweetmeats. It is a powerful antiseptic, delicious and effective in a lozenge, and in tea form is considered a help for old coughs as well as for those patients who have trouble breathing "unless they hold their necks upright." To use elecampane, boil 1 tablespoon of the root in 1 pint of water for ten minutes, then strain and cool the liquid. Use this also to help regulate menstruation and (high) blood acidity.

Garlic   Make a garlic tincture by placing three to four peeled buds in brandy. Steep this in a dark closet for fourteen days. Use several drops at a time, several times a day, for coughs or asthma. Garlic is an exceptional cleanser for the body and has antimicrobial action similar to other antibiotics.

Ginseng   Use ⅛ teaspoon of pure Korean or Siberian ginseng in hot herbal tea or hot water. Ginseng-powder tea frequently eliminates a tenacious cough unresponsive to other medicines.

Honey   Add honey to any herbal drink, or simmer honey and washed and cut lemons in water to prepare a hot honey lemonade. Keep on reusing the old lemon rinds, and add fresh cut lemons and additional honey. This is an effective, inexpensive cough-easing, soothing remedy.

Horehound   The leaves, syrup of the leaves, and candy from the sweet leaves have long been used throughout Europe, especially England, to alleviate coughs.

Tea: Pour 2 cups of boiling water on 2 tablespoons of fresh leaves. Sweeten this with honey. Drink this tea in small amounts (no more than half a cup at a time) several times a day. Large amounts may prove laxative.

Juice: Express juice from the leaves. Use 2 to 3 teaspoons at a time.

Candy: Boil a handful of the fresh plant in 1½ cups of water. Strain the liquid. Use 4 tablespoons of infusion to 2 pounds of brown sugar. Add 1 teaspoon of honey. Boil the mixture for half an hour or so. The candy is finished when a teaspoon hardens when it is dropped into cold water. Pour the mixture into a paper mold, tin mold, or onto a marble slab. Cut it into candy squares when it cools. Gerard considered fresh green horehound leaves and sugar a "singular remedy against coughing and wheezing."

Lemon   See Honey.

Limeflowers (Linden)   Limeflower tea is an old remedy to quiet coughs. The tea is also an effective sleep aid.

Licorice   Add licorice root sticks to any herbal tea to lessen cough.

Mullein   Use dried leaves of this wayside weed for pipe smoking. This is an old remedy to control a hacking or spasmodic cough.

Mustard   Combine mustard seed powder and tepid water to make a mustard plaster or poultice to decongest the chest. Also use mustard in a hot footbath to draw congestion away from the chest.

Onion   Make an onion broth. Cut up a large red onion. Add a pint of cold water, a pinch of salt, and a pat of butter, and simmer until the onion is soft. Place the broth in a hot bowl, and eat it as hot as possible. Minerals from the onion—and the mucilaginous properties of the vegetable—help soothe the inflamed mucous membranes and also induce perspiration. The perspiration helps to reduce the chest congestion and also causes the release of toxins.

Onion-Cherry-Bark-Horehound-Licorice-Honey Remedy   This is best made as an overnight preparation in a large double boiler.

Chop about 2 pounds or 1 quart of onions. Add the onions to the top of a double boiler and cover them with honey. Heat this for a while. Add any, or all, of the following in 1-ounce amounts: cherry bark powder, horehound leaf powder, and licorice powder. After cooking this for at least three to four hours (or overnight), strain out the herbs and press out all juice. Add several ounces of glycerine to the preparation in order to preserve it. Otherwise, store it in the refrigerator. Use a teaspoon at a time to help control cough.

Pine Tree   If you have access to a silver pine tree, make a pillow of the yellow shavings, and sleep on the pillow as an asthma aid.

Peppermint   Use frequent doses of peppermint tea, or 8 to 10 drops of the essence of peppermint (available in the grocery store) in a cup of boiling water. Use 1 teaspoon of the tea at a time.

Slippery Elm   The powder of the bark of the slippery elm is exceptionally soothing for chest complaints. Use a small amount dissolved in water, and add it to any herbal tea. Slippery elm troches (lozenges) are available in health-food stores. Suck on them to relieve tightness in the chest.

Wintergreen   Use oil of wintergreen salve, or wintergreen liniment, to relieve chest tightness and bring blood to the surface of the congested area. Olbas oil is a European herbal combination that contains many effective and soothing oils, including oils of wintergreen and eucalyptus.

CRAMPS AND MUSCLE SPASMS

Arnica   Use arnica lotion or ointment on a cramp or muscle spasm.

Peppermint   Add a scant ½ cup of boiling water to a handful of peppermint leaves to make. wet mash and to release the volatile oil. Apply this as a poultice directly to the area of muscle spasms.

Eucalyptus Oil   Apply it to the muscle spasm.

Olbas Oil or Lotion   This prepared combination of various herbal oils is very effective for massage, sports-induced cramps, and muscle spasms.

Vinegar   Apply compresses of apple cider vinegar to the body on the area of the cramp, spasm, or tension. Use several cups of vinegar in the bathwater.

Vinegar and Honey ★   Use equal amounts of vinegar and honey (1 tablespoon each to a cup of water) for a drink. This may also work for arthritic deposits; it is presumed that it works by distributing locked-in calcium through the entire bloodstream, which lessens chronic cramp. Calcium tablets and vitamin C tablets together are often used by dancers to overcome some nightly cramps.

Water ★   If the cramps are induced by running, it helps to take long, warm sedative baths immediately after jogging, or tennis, or other sport. At night, before bedtime, "walk" in cold water. This often alleviates the frequency of the sports-related nighttime cramp. However, the cramp might be related to posture or to the shoe and the need for a lift in one shoe.

CYSTITIS

Acidophilus ★   Add a capsule to the water and douche. This may help avoid possible yeast infection.

Cranberry Juice Drink lots of cleansing cranberry juice. Douche with cranberry juice and water.

Garlic ★   Drink garlic tea several times a day. Use two to three mashed buds. The body will smell from garlic, but nevertheless, garlic cures and controls this condition. If the strong aroma is objectionable, use the garlic capsule "perles."

DETOXIFICATION ★

There are several ways to detoxify the body. One of the quickest and most effective means is to use the eliminative abilities of the skin to give off stored toxins through perspiration. Another important method is to flush the system with lots of water and cleansing herbal teas. Or a plain, herbal or coffee enema may be used to irrigate the bowel, and laxatives used to cleanse the entire system. Use different detoxification procedures depending on the health problem.

Apple Pectin   Use apple pectin to eliminate metals and radiation from the system.

Basil and Cloves   Use powdered cloves and sweet basil tea, and for long-range body action, combine equal amounts (1 ounce at a time) of powdered sweet basil and powdered cloves into #00 capsules. Use a two-capsule dosage three times a day until *metals* are expelled from the body.

Cayenne Pepper   Use tiny pinches of cayenne pepper and

water and apple cider vinegar and honey, or apple cider vinegar and water drinks, to eliminate the smell of too much chlorine after swimming in a pool.

Coffee   Use pure, undiluted coffee as a detoxifying enema to extract poisons, or to normalize the body. This is a *very* strong action.

Fennel   Crush several tablespoons, simmer them in boiling water, and steep and strain the liquid. Use it as hot or cold tea, in a vaporizer, and in bathwater, to withdraw toxins.

Hayflower   Make up a strong tea of hayflower, or use prepared Swiss extract and add it to bathwater or a foot or arm bath, to withdraw toxins from the system. This is great to do right before a cold appears to be coming on.

Oatmeal   Apply a paste of oatmeal, or oatmeal and banana paste, to withdraw foreign objects from a cut or wound. I alternate this paste with salad-oil "compresses," for embedded splinters and can often just squeeze them out.

Oatstraw   Like hayflower, oatstraw has strong detoxifying abilities. Use it in compresses, as a poultice, or in full or partial baths.

Peach   Simmer several peach pits to achieve a red-colored tea. Store it in the refrigerator. Use the tea in small doses to help pull drug effects from the body. Use it for worms. Use it as an enema for detoxification purposes. Make a tincture for future use. Use 15 drops in a glass of water.

Salt   Add between a cup to a pound of common coarse table salt to bathwater to give the effect of seawater and help detoxify the body. This is useful after a hard day in a city or after an evening of smoking or drinking. Salt can also be rubbed on the body to create additional circulation and a feeling of well-being.

Salt and Baking Soda   Use a combination of salt and baking soda in the bath to offset the effect of minor X-ray or radiation exposure.

DIARRHEA

Persistent diarrhea calls for a visit to a health professional.

Agrimony   Control bowel looseness with tea made from agrimony stem, leaves, or flowers, Agrimony is a table tea in France.

Barley   Cooked barley or barley water is an excellent infant diarrhea aid.

Blackberry   The bark or roots are quite astringent and can help against diarrhea. For tea, use 2 tablespoons in 3 cups of water and simmer it until the tea is reduced to 2 cups. The dose is 1 to 2 tablespoons at a time, up to four times a day—or more if needed. Blackberry syrup or blackberry extract, available in many food departments or health-food stores, may be used as a basis for tea.

Blueberry   Combine a tablespoon of blueberry extract with 4 tablespoons of water, and drink the liquid every two hours to control diarrhea. Make this extract during the season by steeping blueberries or huckleberries in brandy for two weeks and straining out the berries.

Limeflowers (Linden)   These flowers are sedative and anti-spasmodic. Use them as tea.

Nutmeg   An ⅛ teaspoon of freshly grated nutmeg is always acceptable with other herbal teas for aroma, and for its slight binding ability.

Peppermint   Use peppermint tea to allay spasms, diarrhea, or digestive disturbance. For children's diarrhea, bruise a handful of fresh peppermint, add a tablespoon of water to create a paste, and apply it directly to the abdomen and navel area. This will help to control the diarrhea.

Rice   Cooked rice is useful in controlling irritable diarrhea.

Yellow Pond Lily   This may be useful while backpacking. Shave several 5-inch pieces of root and steep in cold water. Simmer this for five minutes. Steep the pieces again for several hours, then strain them. This preparation may also be used for sore-throat gargles, vaginal douche, or skin inflammations.

DIGESTIVE FLATULENCE AND INDIGESTION (SEE ALSO *NAUSEA.*)

Despite varying symptoms, many digestive problems may stem from body imbalance, hasty eating, wrong nutrition, or general stress. Some health professionals suggest faulty digestion can sometimes be helped by adding hydrochloric acid tablets to the daily diet (see Vinegar, below). The following is a rundown of herbs that can relieve many *temporary* digestive inconveniences and may, with improvements in eating, chewing well, and stress management, relieve some chronic conditions. Since persistent digestive problems may be an indication of other systemic conditions, consult a health professional.

Anise   Drink bruised anise seed tea, or add drops of anisette liqueur to alleviate wind and colic.

Caraway   Drink bruised caraway seed tea, or prepare a cold infusion to control infant or adult flatulence. Caraway julep: Bruise 2 tablespoons of the seed in 2 cups of cold water. Steep it for six hours, then strain. Dose: 1 to 3 teaspoons, depending on the age of child.

Cayenne ★   Cayenne pepper is sharp on the tongue but

benign and effective for most digestive complaints. Add a few grains (up to ⅛ teaspoon) to chamomile, peppermint, or other suggested digestive teas to relieve the feeling of discomfort.

Centaury The root of this flower was always used by the herbalist Kunzle to overcome heartburn.

Chamomile ★ Sweet, apple-scented, and benign, chamomile tea is the tea to use to control intestinal spasms. Use it also as an enema and for an abdominal poultice.

Cinnamon The aroma and the volatile oil of this bark are valuable assets in indigestion and flatulence control. Add it to other herbal teas, and use it with any seeds or cloves.

Cloves Make a tea with 1 tablespoon to a pint of boiling water, or add bruised cloves to other herbal teas.

Coriander Use this interesting seed in cooking, or add it crushed to various compound powder-drinks.

Cumin Combine it with other herbs in digestive teas.

Dill Bruise a teaspoon of the seeds and add that to half a cup of boiled water. Steep and strain. This is a marvelous carminative (eliminates gas) for infants.

Fennel ★ This is another outstanding herb to ease stomachache. Soak bruised fennel seeds in cold water (see caraway julep) or in hot tea (cool it first) for infant colic or digestive unease.

Ginger ★ In India, Europeans who suffer from indigestion are given ginger tea instead of regular tea. Ginger tea is stimulant and carminative, and therefore useful in dealing with infant colic or flatulence.

Juniper Berries ★ A berry cure for indigestion and flatulence: Eat and carefully chew four berries on the first day, five on the second day, six on the third day, seven on the fourth day, up to twelve berries a day. Next, work backward from twelve until only five are taken in a day. The husks may either be swallowed or discarded.

Nutmeg   A tiny amount of grated fresh nutmeg may be added to any herbal tea to help relieve flatulence.

Peppermint ★   Peppermint leaves, peppermint essence, or drops of peppermint oil are invaluable aids in all digestive discomforts, including diarrhea. Spearmint may also be used for flatulence.

Valerian   The herb is useful for occasional stress or nervous attacks, for nervous headache, or for flatulent indigestion, but should *not* be used on a steady, daily basis. Use a small pill, or a tiny amount of refrigerated fresh valerian juice (German import).

Vinegar ★   Small amounts of apple cider vinegar and water will often relieve indigestion and heartburn. If the treatment works, it frequently indicates that the body has a shortage of the acids needed in the digestive system. Apple cider vinegar and honey (1 tablespoon each) plus a cup of water may also be used once to several times a day to help rebalance the body.

DIURETIC (INCREASING THE SECRETION OF URINE)

Apple ★   An apple-juice fast, preferably with organic apple juice, will cleanse the system and stimulate the kidneys and the liver.

Broom (Cytisus scoparius)   Dried or fresh twigs of broom contain an alkaloid which will be released in a decoction. The tea will increase the flow of urine.

Celery Celery seeds act on the kidneys. Bruise and add 3 tablespoons of the seeds to a pint of brandy or red wine. Steep them for several days. Dosage: a tablespoon at a time with 2 tablespoons of water, three times a day. This celery-seed brandy is also useful for flatulence.

Corn Silk Make tea from the yellow strands of "silk" beneath the husk of corn. Corn silk is a wonderful and effective diuretic.

Grapes Eat grapes freely to induce free flow of urine from the system. That is why certain wines are so effective as a mild diuretic.

Juniper ★ Juniper berries eaten in dried form—as well as juniper berries steeped in wine or combined with several other herbs—produce a powerful diuretic action.

½ tablespoon juniper berries
½ tablespoon dandelion root
½ tablespoon broom tops
1 pint water

Boil all the ingredients on a low flame until the water reduces to ½ pint. Strain the liquid and put it in a labeled jar. Drink 2 tablespoons three times a day.

Onions ★ Raw onions increase the flow of urine. They are, therefore, excellent in a raw tomato, onion, and garlic salad (add lemon juice and oil). This combination will not only increase the flow of urine, but eliminate toxins from the system. It is excellent at the onset of a cold.

Parsley ★ Eat crushed parsley, add it to other juices from extractor, or make parsley soup, or drink parsley herbal juice, available in some health-food stores. Parsley can also be used cooked with juniper berries.

EARS

Check persistent or intense earaches with a health professional. This is particularly important for infants as a serious infection may lead to a mastoid bone infection or lifelong hearing defect.

Caraway   Heat an unsliced bread loaf in the oven. Throw away the crust and pound together the soft bread and a handful of bruised caraway seeds. Add some hot brandy and apply the paste as a hot poultice to the ear or any other inflammation.

Chamomile   Steep the flowers in boiling water. Strain out the water, and apply the hot flowers in a cloth for alleviation of the earache.

Garlic   An old country remedy: Peel the skin from the bud. Cut the bud into the right size to fit the outer ear canal if it is sore or inflamed. Apply the garlic encased in gauze to prevent blistering.

(Wild) Ginger   Ginger has antimicrobial properties. The Meskwaki Indians crushed and simmered the root as an ear poultice.

Mullein   The yellow flowers of mullein provide an excellent earache oil which relieves internal and external pain and ear eczema. Steep the flowers in sunlight for twenty-one days. Strain out the oil. Add additional mullein flowers and repeat the process several times. Mullein oil is available from reputable homoeopathic pharmacies.

Onion   Roast the onion to modify its acrid oil, then apply it hot to the ear to relieve pain and control discharge from the ear.

Yarrow Winnebago Indians steeped the whole yarrow plant and poured the liquid into the aching ear. Control the liquid by using absorbent cotton.

ECZEMA

Since eczema is a systemic health problem, it responds to a series of nutritional, herbal, friction, washes approach. These include addition of walking outdoors, exercise, water and juice drinking program, possible water-juice-herb-drink-fast, and a continuous series of stimulating dry friction or salt bath rubs, all these to stimulate sluggish elimination of toxic wastes from the system.

Another integral part of eczema control is addition of various nutritional supplements, especially vitamins B for stress, vitamin A, and the fatty acids from various oils, or wheat germ, or various salad oils. Use herb lotions and a series of foot and hand baths instead of topical drugs that turn the skin lesions back into the body.

Aloe Vera gel Open up leaf of house plant, aloe vera, and spread on topically.

Blackberry leaf tea Use as topical lotion.

Oatmeal Take baths in blended particles, or Aveeno brand colloidal oatmeal. This may cause the bath to be slippery, so make sure you have a hand grip and mat in the bath. This will reduce any itching.

Eczema Foot and Hand Bath Extract
Maurice Messegue, the French herbalist, in his book *Of men and Plants,* claims the following recipe for plant extract and continuous 8-minute hand and foot baths has a ninety-eight percent cure rate:

Boil one quart of water. Cool.

Steep handful of *artichoke* leaves, *elecampane* flowers and leaves, *great Burdock* leaves, *buttercup* flowers and leaves, *greater celandine* leaves, *chicory* roots and tips, *broom* flowers, *lavender* flowers, *nettle* leaves (fresh if possible).

Soak the leaves, flowers and roots for four to five hours. Strain and pour into labeled bottle. Store for up to eight days in refrigerator.

To Use: Boil 2 quarts of water. Cool for five minutes.

Add one cup of the above plant extract to the water.

Soak feet in eight-minute foot bath before breakfast. Use hot as possible.

Soak hands for eight-minute hand bath before dinner. Use hot as possible.

This material may be used again for additional baths, but it is *not* to be heated or boiled again.

EYES

Apple Roast an apple in the oven and apply the pulp—as warm as you can comfortably stand—to relieve inflamed or tired eyes.

Borage Eat young borage leaves in a salad, and use strong borage tea to strengthen the eyes.

Cabbage The ancient Greeks used fresh white cabbage juice (with tiny amounts of honey added) to relieve sore or in-flamed, moist, running eyes. For runny eyes in infants, cleanse the eyes every half hour with warm water. Bruise fresh cabbage leaves to a soft pulp and apply a cabbage pack to the closed eyes. This will tend to increase the flow for a few days, but will cure the condition after a very short while thereafter.

My grandmother's cure for inflamed and sick eyes: Wash the eyes every morning with fasting saliva. Add saliva to a small amount of green or grey (pure) clay, and apply it as poultice to the closed eyes. Meanwhile, boil cabbage leaves and dip a cloth into the cabbage water. Apply the wet cloth over the clay pack. Wash the eyes off with warm water when the clay dries. Repeat this each morning for as long as necessary.

Chamomile Chamomile tea compresses and chamomile tea rinses are eye easing, and applications can be repeated as often as necessary.

Cucumber Pink eyes, sunburn, and eyestrain may all be relieved by application of cooling and refreshing cucumber slices to the closed eyes.

Eyebright ★ For simple inflammation and bloodshot eyes, steep a handful of fresh or dried eyebright in a pint of brandy. Strain the liquid after two weeks. Combine 30 drops of tincture with 4 tablespoons of rosewater (another eye-easer). Use this mixture several times a day on pads over the eyes.

Use cool fresh eyebright tea eye *wash* daily (one tablespoon to cup of boiled water) to strengthen the eyes and help control many eye problems.

This ancient folk medicine is very effective.

Fennel ★ For eyewash, add half a teaspoon of fennel powder (made from crushed and blended fennel seeds) to 2½ ounces of clear cold water. Strain the liquid and use it as a lotion for almost any eye problem. Several old histories report instances where monks used fennel root for control of cataracts, but unlike folk medicine recipes, which are handed down from family to family, from century to century, this appears to be hearsay.

Goldenseal For a lotion, steep half a teaspoon of goldenseal root powder in a cup of just-boiled water. Cool the liquid. Make sure the powder is thoroughly dissolved. This was used by many midwestern Indian tribes and early American settlers, and later by Seventh Day Adventists. Keep the eyes closed, and apply the lotion with absorbent cotton.

Rosewater Rosewater is a simple and surprisingly effective eye-easer. Use it on compresses for inflamed eyes.

Tansy   Tansy tea is said to be effective for eye inflammation or sty compress. Always discard the gauze used on sties, to control possible contagion.

Thyme   Dioscorides, the great Greek physician, wrote that thyme added to food helps overcome dimness of sight.

Witch Hazel   Use witch hazel compresses for relief of sore, red, strained, or inflamed eyes. Use it on closed eyes.

Yarrow   The Blackfoot Indians used an infusion of yarrow leaf and yarrow flower for an eye wash.

FEVER

Add huge quantities of cool water to the diet!

Apple   Apple water is excellent for feverish patients. Prepare it by slicing three washed, unpeeled apples; simmer them in very little water until they are soft. Strain the apples through a fine strainer or cloth, and add a washed piece of lemon for flavor. Drink it cold.

Barley Water   Barley water has been used from earliest civilizations to assist patients in high fever. Because it has no irritating properties, it is especially helpful where either the chest lining or intestinal lining is inflamed. For the recipe, see "Colds."

Cayenne   Cayenne pepper is used by American Indians, Mexican Indians, and various African tribes to cure all kinds of fever. Add a pinch or more of the pepper to any herbal drink.

Fenugreek   Drink unstrained fenugreek, lemon juice, and honey tea. This will soothe and nourish the body, and help to reduce the fever.

Ginseng   Ginseng powder will help to regulate the body

temperature. It is also a body-restorer and alterative. Use as the Chinese do—add it to chicken soup to help restore ill patients to normal health.

Grapes   Grapes and greatly diluted grape juice are very restorative, and act on the kidneys to increase the flow of urine. This is useful in reducing fever.

Lemon   Lemon juice and lemon drinks have long been used in the Mediterranean area to control minor and major fever attacks. Take a fresh, unpeeled washed lemon, cut it into thin slices, add 3 large cups of water, and simmer the slices in a nonaluminum pot. Reduce the juice to 1 cup, strain it, and give it to the patient. Lemon is a refrigerant (cooling) plant: It is useful in all inflammatory and feverish conditions. It may be added to the barley water.

Raspberry Vinegar   Use fresh raspberries and crush them into apple cider vinegar. Drink this diluted with water for an exceptionally refreshing drink during any fever attacks or for a sore throat. If a good raspberry jam is available, it may be used diluted in water, and added to the vinegar.

Rice   Cook rice with lots of water and drink the strained water. This is a nutritious drink for feverish conditions or for an inflammation of the lungs or bowels.

Strawberries   Pour water on crushed, bruised strawberries for a somewhat laxative, refreshing, cooling, and purifying drink.

Water   Plain cold water will quickly reduce a fever within the body. Sponge the patient with cool water, and briskly wipe each area as sponged. This cools the body and increases circulation. For high fevers, use a cool to cold enema to reduce internal body heat. Flush the body by drinking large quantities of pure water and pure lemon, grape, or raspberry drinks.

FLU PREVENTION

See Vinegar of the Four Thieves, *cayenne-vinegar-salt preparation and cinnamon preparation*.
Also my grandmother would prepare this combination
tea:

> handful wormwood
> handful sage
> handful alpine speedwell
> handfull licorice root
> 1   pint of boiling water

Add boiling water. Steep the mixture for half an hour.
Take a spoonful every half hour, or sip it morning and
evening. The recovery time was usually two days. ★

GLANDS

Apple Cider Vinegar   Dip cloths in the vinegar, wring out, and
use them as compresses on swollen glands. For neck glands,
cover the first wet cloth with a larger wool sock so the area can
heat up from within.

Burdock   Apply bruised or wet bruised burdock leaves as a
poultice to reduce glandular swellings.

Cumin   Soak bruised cumin seeds in ninety-proof alcohol or
brandy. This makes an excellent "warming" liniment to
overcome congestion in any area.

Fennel   Apply the bruised plant on glandular swelling.

Flaxseed   Extract the valuable and healing linseed oil by
pouring boiling water over several tablespoons of the seeds.

Encase the seed mash in a clean cloth, and apply it to the swollen area (or sore throat or congested chest) in poultice form. The crushed seed can also be used for poultices.

Ginseng ★   The root acts as a body and glandular balancer. While I was in Korea I learned a lot of uses for this unusual herb. Chew the fresh or dried root, or add ⅛ of a teaspoon of the white powder or extract to hot herbal tea.

Ginseng energizes the entire body because it stimulates the adrenals and the spleen. Use small amounts of ginseng powder to regulate temperature imbalances during hot weather and during menopause.

I have discovered that a really small amount of ginseng from reputable sources will help control most hayfever and sinus attacks.

HAIR TONICS

Use apple cider vinegar rinse water to cleanse hair of soap. Prepare a strong tea of chamomile for a light hair rinse. Burdock leaf tea cleanses the system and helps give the hair additional shine from within, and may be used for very cleansing hair rinse also. Nettle juice cleanses the system and provides help for lackluster skin and hair. Rhubarb root tea rinse will lighten light brown or faded blond hair. Sage tea will stimulate hair growth.

HEADACHE

As with many other body symptoms, headaches can be traced to different causes. In addition to polluted environment, minute gas leaks in the home, fluorescent lights in home or office, neck and shoulder tension, eyestrain, grinding of the teeth, toothaches, and postural eccentricities, headaches can also be brought on by such things as a cold, fever, or other internal malfunctioning. Chronic headaches, of course, should be brought to the attention of a health professional.

Very often a neutral-temperature full bath will take away a tension headache. If your area of tension is concentrated about the neck and shoulders, apply a steaming hot towel to the neck and shoulders during the bath.

Another water remedy is the hot footbath. The addition of mustard powder to the bath will draw blood away from the head area to the feet, and thus relieve the headache.

The following teas are extremely useful in clearing the head or alleviating digestive distress causing a headache:

For General Headache Relief Cold balm (melissa), basil, cayenne pepper (a few grains added to other teas), chamomile flowers, ginger, (sweet) marjoram, parsley, peppermint, rosemary, sage. Use garlic buds in salad to clear headache. Use a lavender oil or water or lotion on the forehead. A tiny valerian discote (pill) will also relieve nervous tension.

HEART

> **Anyone who thinks he or she may have any sort of heart problem should consult a physician at once. The herbal aids below should be used only after approval by your physician.**

Asparagus Asparagus shoots and roots are very diuretic and can help with edema caused by heart trouble.

(Wild) Cherry Use tea made from the bark, or use wild cherry syrup added to tea to help nervous palpitations of the heart. This tea can also be used for a spasmodic cough.

Garlic and Onions   A recent abstract in *Nutrition Reviews* indicates positive findings in the essential oil found in both garlic and onion which "are reported to lower serum cholesterol levels and stimulate fibrinolytic activity."

Hawthorn Berries   Several European firms make up an excellent syrup and extract and fresh juice of hawthorn berries for use as a heart tonic.

Lemon Juice   Lemon juice plus water has sedative action and can help sedate nervous palpitations.

Rosemary   Rosemary is both quieting and tonic, and may help the kidneys reduce edema caused by a malfunctioning heart.

HEMORRHOIDS AND SUPPOSITORIES

Cut a red potato into a cigar-shaped suppository and insert it. Melt 2 ounces of cocoa butter on top of a double boiler, and stir in 2 tablespoons of finely powdered witch hazel, yellow dock, or bayberry (all astringent herbs). When they are in a pliable condition roll these into cigar-shaped inserts. Harden them in the refrigerator. Cocoa butter melts at body temperature. Check into watery therapy irrigation and foot massage at acupuncture contact points for additional aid. (See also Suppositories in Section Three.)

HIGH BLOOD PRESSURE–
LOW BLOOD PRESSURE

These two conditions are systemic symptoms that must be appraised from a holistic point of view. Nonetheless, it is interesting to note that one herb—garlic—is said to have a beneficial effect on both these conditions and that the eating of citrus fruits is negative. Yellow dock, garlic, and ginger are folk remedies that may be explored in addition to standard medical treatment. Both these ailments call for the advice of a physician—even if you only suspect that there may be a blood-pressure problem.

(Yellow) Dock   Make up dock seed or dock herb tea and drink several cups a day for high blood pressure.

Garlic   This is an old and very effective folk medicine. It sometimes takes only a few days of raw garlic "tea" or raw garlic-carrot "sandwiches," or high garlic content salads to bring down high blood pressure. Low blood pressure also responds to the garlic intake, but the garlic may be taken in capsule form instead of the raw form.

Ginger   Ginger tea seems to help people with low blood pressure, especially B_{12}. Make sure the vitamin E supplements are accurate in quantity—not too high. That ancient Greek standby, oxymel—the combination of vinegar, honey, and water—is also of use in low blood pressure stabilization. Use 1 tablespoon of apple cider vinegar and 1 of honey to 1 cup of water; drink this freely during each day.

Note: Anyone who thinks he or she has abnormal blood pressure should consult a health professional, but in any case I recommend regular diagnostic checkups.

INFANTS

See details on chamomile (useful for teething and colic), linden (lime-blossoms) (useful for sleep aid), caraway julep and fennel water and other herbs useful for digestion, flatulence, diarrhea, constipation, first aid and so on. Do not use uncooked honey as a food for infants up to one year of age.

It is valuable to keep Syrup of Ipecac (available from the drugstore) in the home medicine chest as it is a staple in overcoming some accidental poisonings. For emergencies have local Poison Control Center telephone number in accessible spot. *You should be very careful in giving infants compound herbal mixtures,* especially if you aren't absolutely sure of the contents of prepared herbal teas. There were recent reported infant fatalities from the use of excellent mixtures which contained buckthorn, another than contained senna, both effective laxatives, but too powerful for infants and children.

INFECTED SORES

See *Inflammation* and *Boils.*

Peach   Simmer several pits, wash the infected area with red tea, and apply the peach pit compresses. For tendencies for infection, make up peach pit tincture during peach season. Use 15–30 drops in a glass of water. Soak cloth in water and apply.

INFLAMMATION

Comfrey   Use comfrey root or comfrey leaf tea compresses to reduce inflammation. For inflamed sores, use comfrey ointment or comfrey lotion.

Plantain   Wrap a bruised wet plantain leaf around inflamed area. Keep it wet by enclosing it in plastic or by wrapping it with a larger dry cloth. I have known plantain to work on infected finger sores unresponsive to antibiotic ointment.

Vinegar   Use apple cider vinegar compresses to reduce heat and inflammation of bruises.

Witch Hazel   Apply large soaking-wet witch hazel compresses to swellings and inflammations on almost any part of the body.

ITCHING

Apple Cider Vinegar ★   Add 2 cups of apple cider vinegar to bathwater to relieve itching, or apply full strength apple cider directly to the area of the itch, except near the eyes or the genitals. Douche with diluted apple cider vinegar to relieve itching caused by *Trichomonas vaginitis.*

Anise   Anise oil destroys lice and similar insects. Apply it directly to the area of itching, or make up an anise ointment.

Ointment   Bruise a handful of anise seeds, and add them to either wheat germ oil, vitamin E oil, avocado oil, pure lanolin, or lard. Bake this for two hours in an oven. Then strain out the charred seeds. Apply the result to the itching area or to the area with lice. Check first for skin sensitivity.

Burdock   It is said that homeopathic tincture of burdock seeds in dose of 10 to 30 drops in 2 tablespoons of cold water used from several weeks to several months will overcome many chronic skin diseases. I have also read reports of success in treating psoriasis with burdock.

Dock (Yellow Curled)   Boil the root of yellow curled dock in vinegar until it softens. Mix the pulp with vegetable oil or any of the above-mentioned oils, and apply the mixture to the skin to alleviate an old skin condition. The diluted homeopathic tincture may also be used in this way. Fresh dock leaves will help relieve the itch of poison ivy.

Juniper   An ointment of juniper wood oil ("juniper tar") and yellow wax *(Unguentum olei cadini),* has been used by herbalists and physicians to heal eczema and psoriasis skin sores.

Lemon Juice   Fresh squeezed lemon juice will relieve itching. Use it diluted, on genital areas.

Oatmeal ★   Use either colloidal oatmeal from the drugstore, or uncooked blended oatmeal in bathwater, or add a small amount of water to get a paste consistency, and apply the oatmeal to the skin to overcome itching. Oatmeal paste or baths relieve the itch of poison ivy, hives, and other allergic reactions.

Yogurt ★   Dilute several tablespoons of yogurt or acidophilus tablets in a pint of warm water. Use this as a douche to relieve internal itching from yeast infection. Also add yogurt or acidophilus to the diet to prevent yeast infections.

JOINTS

Arnica   Use Arnica compresses, lotion, or liniment on the areas of joint pain.

Ginger   Use ginger compresses or ginger foot soaks to relieve pain.

Eucalyptus   Prepare a strong tea with ¼ cup of eycalyptus leaves and several quarts of water. Add the tea to the bathwater, and soak in the bath to relieve pain.

Olbas Oil   Use olbas prepared oil for massages or rubs. It contains several heat-producing, pain-relieving herbs.

Onions   Briefly roast a half dozen onions, and place them directly on the painful or swollen joint. Tie them to the body with a large elastic bandage.

Vinegar   Apply apple cider vinegar compresses. Add apple cider vinegar to bathwater. Drink apple cider vinegar and honey (½ tablespoon of each) in a cup of water several times a day.

KIDNEY CONGESTION

Asparagus   Steam asparagus, or use a good brand of canned asparagus. The minerals and "asparagin" stimulate the kidney and contribute a special smell to the urine almost immediately after eating.

Cayenne Pepper ★   Add a few grains of red pepper to any hot herbal tea for restorative and tonic digestive action. This then helps the kidney to perform in a more normal fashion.

Parsley   Parsley tea and parsley soup will increase the flow of urine.

LAXATIVES

Fennel   Fennel seed powder will relieve the griping action of stronger cathartics, such as senna.

Licorice   A famous English laxative (Compound Powder of Licorice) uses licorice, senna, fennel, and sugar.

Psyllium   Swallow the dried seeds, or mix the seeds with juice and drink it down. The seeds expand and decrease the density of the feces.

Purslane   The whole plant is slightly laxative.

Rhubarb   This root is both peculiar and valuable in medicine, as it combines gentle laxative action and astringent action. Therefore, it has often been used in children's bowel complaints and to sometimes overcome the causes of diarrhea by evacuating toxic materials from the lower bowel. It comes in pill form and also as Aromatic Syrup of Rhubarb, which is prepared with small amounts of cloves, cinnamon, nutmeg, and rhubarb root powder. Purchase this syrup from a drugstore, and use it as directed.

Senna This herb is a powerful laxative. It is used by many radiologists prior to exploratory X-rays to cleanse the system of fecal matter. The griping action (intermittent severe pains in the bowel) of senna can be controlled by a pinch of ginger or fennel.

Sweet Flag This valuable medicinal root, also known as calamus, is readily available in the outdoors. For digestive problems, constipation, or restorative purposes, make a gruel of small quantities of the powdered or crushed root, wheat flour, and milk. Sweeten the gruel with honey.

Kneipp's Tonic Laxative

2   tablespoons powdered fennel
2   tablespoons (crushed) juniper berries
1   tablespoon fenugreek
1   teaspoon aloe powder

Mix the ingredients in dry form. Put the mixture in a closed, lidded jar. Keep it in a dry place.

Use 1 teaspoon of the combination and add it to 6 ounces of water. Simmer this for fifteen minutes. Drink it warm or cold, with or without sugar.

Dose:

Weak: Divide 1 cup over the course of two to three days. Or the strong form: Take 2 cupfuls in a row. Take them at night before going to bed. It may take as long as twelve to thirteen hours to work in its weak state, but according to Father Kneipp there is no uncomfortable feeling with this compound laxative. Here the aloe powder has the strongest laxative action.

Since aloe causes bowel spasms (griping), it is imperative to use it with fennel, juniper berries, and fenugreek.

Note: There are several excellent prepared laxatives on the market: Among them are Inner-Clean and Swiss-Kriss. They are mild, effective, and nonhabit-forming.

LIVER

There are many foods and herbs that stimulate the liver and bile action. Others will help reduce liver inflammation.

Apples ★   Eating fresh apples will stimulate a sluggish liver. Apples may be used for a monofast to cleanse the entire body.

Beets ★   Add a small amount of fresh extracted beet juice to the daily diet to slowly cleanse the liver.

Asparagus ★   The roots and shoots of asparagus have a stimulating action on both the kidney and liver, and increase the flow of liquids from the body.

Burdock   Burdock leaf packs are useful on the inflamed liver area. Alternate them with castor oil packs or peppermint and cinnamon packs.

Castor Oil   Apply continuous and frequent castor oil packs for a healing and detoxifying action on an inflamed liver.

Celery ★   Eat lots of celery.

Centaury ★   The whole herb is a bitter tonic. Drink centaury tea before meals to stimulate liver and bile action.

Chicory ★   Its leaves and root are stimulating for the liver.

Coffee   A pure coffee enema has a strong cleansing action, and is a liver-detoxifying aid.

Dandelion   Young dandelion leaves in early spring and two-year-old root coffee and fresh expressed dandelion juice have a stimulating action on the liver.

Lemon Juice ★   Lemon juice and water promote bile activity within the body.

Peppermint   Make up a strong tea of peppermint leaves; add concentrated cinnamon tea, and use this as a poultice directly on the inflamed liver area.

Prune   Prune whip before breakfast is a fantastic cleanser for the liver: Cut up 6 to 8 medium-to-large prunes. Whip up a half pint of heavy cream, add the prunes, chopped, and eat this first thing in the morning. Then do not eat breakfast, and try to avoid lunch.

Rosemary   Drink rosemary tea to stimulate a sluggish liver.

MEMORY

Ginseng ★   Add a few grains of ginseng powder to daily herbal teas as a memory aid and stimulant. Special double-blind tests have shown the memory action of adult students to be increased with small amounts of ginseng in the diet.

Gotu Kola   Poor memory is said to be revived with small amounts of this herb in your tea several days in a row. However, do not use this tea continuously or in great amounts.

Rosemary   Ancient use of this herb included drinking tea to "comfort the brain" and "refresh the memory."

MENSTRUATION

TOO PROFUSE

Carrot ★   Grate and dry carrots, and eat one piece at a time, several times a day, as a potent aid to regulate menstruation. Grate about a pound from the heaviest part of the carrot. Dry it on paper in the sun for a week or two until it shrivels up into small pieces.

Cayenne Pepper ★   Add a few grains of the herb to any herbal tea of your choice. Cayenne has the power to regulate bleeding within and without the body, and may have some effect on the menstrual flow.

Cinnamon Bark   Utilize a few drops of the diluted cinnamon bark tincture to help control a profuse flow.

Lemon Juice ★   Drink diluted lemon juice during the menstrual period. It not only serves to cleanse the entire system, but has an indirect effect on bleeding. Lemon juice can also be used as a styptic to stop external bleeding from cuts.

Lentil   Gerard says lentils "are singular good to stay the menses."

(Red) Raspberry   Make a strong tea of red raspberry leaves to control an excessive flow. This herb is also an excellent female tonic during pregnancy.

Shepherd's Purse   This is a great herb to stop hemorrhaging in any part of the body. Infuse a handful in a pint of boiling water. Drink the tea warm if possible. Use 2 cups three times a day (6 cups). Also douche with the same strength brew. Also apply a shepherd's purse tea compress to the pelvic area during excessive flow.

Thyme   Drink a half cup of strong thyme tea each morning and evening to control excessive menstrual flow. Apply a cold thyme tea compress to the pelvic area.

TO PROMOTE DELAYED MENSTRUATION

Angelica   Drink angelica root tea several times a day. To prepare it, bruise 2 tablespoons of root, simmer it in 2 cups of boiling water for fifteen minutes, and strain.

Balm   Release the volatile oil of garden melissa plant by steeping 2 tablespoons of the whole plant in a cup of boiling water. Strain the tea and drink it hot several times a day.

Basil   Fresh sweet basil is an old folk remedy for delayed menstruation. To prepare, use 1 tablespoon of basil to a cup of boiling water; steep, strain.

Beets ★   Many nutritionists and herbalists consider the fresh, raw beet or beet juice or beet powder an invaluable aid in regulating all menstrual problems.

Dill   Release the valuable oil in the seeds by bruising 1 teaspoon of them and steeping them in boiling water; strain this and drink the tea.

Elecampane   Gently simmer the clean root—1 tablespoon to a pint of water. After ten minutes, withdraw the liquid from the heat and let it cool. Strain it and drink 1 to 2 tablespoons of it several times a day.

Fennel   Frequently drink hot tea prepared from bruised fennel seeds simmered for five minutes in boiling water and strained.

Marigold   The petals of the pot marigold (calendula) may be used in tablespoon doses. It has long been considered an aid in regulating monthly flow.

FOR PAINFUL PERIODS

Catnip   Drink catnip tea each morning and evening during the period. Prepare this tea with leaf sprays and flowers, and use 1 teaspoon to a cup of boiling water.

Chamomile   Chamomile tea will gently relieve menstrual spasms.

Peppermint ★   Peppermint tea is a digestive aid and will ease the feeling of bloat and pain during the period.

Strawberry   Tea of strawberry leaves taken over a long period of time will eventually regulate menstrual flow.

MOUTH AND GUMS

Comfrey ★   Comfrey mouthwash, comfrey tea bags, or comfrey ointment will help heal many mouth abrasions. After tooth extraction, put a few drops of boiling water on a comfrey tea bag—just enough to wet it slightly. Tap some goldenseal root powder on the damp bag, and place the bag over the extraction. The combination serves to reduce the swelling, pain, and bleeding.

Goldenseal ★   See the above notation. Goldenseal and myrrh are an excellent combination for most mouth problems, including canker sores and gum infections. The herbs may be used alone or together and make an admirable and effective poultice. The combination may help tighten loose teeth.

Myrrh ★   Tincture of myrrh may be used as an antiseptic and healing mouthwash or, combined with a small amount of goldenseal root, as a mouthwash or poultice.

Peach   Peach pit tea is useful for mouth infections. Rinse out the mouth with the hot tea three times a day (without swallowing it).

Oak Bark ★   Oak bark is strongly astringent and may be used to contract the tissues when this is necessary. Use oak bark rinses and, between the teeth, oak bark packings to help draw newly loosened teeth together. This should be continued on a night-by-night basis until the gums and teeth are in a normal relationship again.

NAUSEA
(See also Digestive Flatulence and Indigestion.)

(Sweet) Basil   Bruised aromatic leaves of sweet basil act as a powerful tonic and will help reduce nausea.

Ginger ★   Add a pinch of ginger to other teas to help reduce nausea. Ginger compress on the head (made with the mild tea) will help relieve headache due to nausea.

Goldenseal   Drink a mild tea of goldenseal and honey immediately upon rising to offset the nausea of pregnancy. Prepare the tea with a pinch of goldenseal powder in a cup of just-boiled water; add a small amount of honey to it to overcome the bitter taste.

Peppermint ★   Reduce a feeling of nausea with a cup of hot, aromatic peppermint tea. A pinch of basil and/or ginger may also be added. I also like a pinch of bruised cloves and/or some cinnamon.

NEURALGIA

Allspice   Allspice berries give off a heady aroma of cinnamon, cloves, pepper, and juniper berries. To use the berries for rheumatic pain, boil them and prepare a thick paste from them (the medicinal values are in the rind). Place the paste in a folded cloth and apply that as a poultice to the area of the pain.

Celery   Drink celery juice, or brew up celery tea and drink it several times a day to help alleviate some forms of sciatica or neuralgia. The celery may also be added to other greens when you prepare freshly extracted juice.

Chamomile   Stuff small bags with chamomile (several tea bags will do). Infuse them in ¼ cup boiling water, and apply them as hot as possible to the inflammation or neuralgic pain. This is quite helpful in facial neuralgia, too.

Coltsfoot   Soak a handful of dried coltsfoot leaves in boiling water and use them on back and loin neuralgic pains for a soothing poultice. Coltsfoot leaf tincture may also be prepared in advance. Add a few drops of the tincture to boiling water. Dip a cloth into the hot water, wring it out, and apply it as a compress to the area of pain.

Horseradish   Scrape horseradish and apply the scrapings directly to the face to quickly relieve facial neuralgia. If the scrapings are held in the hand, the hand will also become numb and white.

Juniper Berries   Apply the bruised juniper berries to rheumatic or neuralgic swellings or to any painful area for effective and lasting relief.

Lemon   The Chinese cut and rub fresh lemons on a neuralgic area to relieve the pain.

Peppermint Oil The Chinese produce a crystalline oil of peppermint (Po ho yo) that is very high in menthol. This can be rubbed over the neuralgic area, facial tic douloureux, or for neuralgic toothache.

NERVOUSNESS

Cumin Tiny amounts of cumin oil (2 to 3 drops of oil to a drop of sugar) can help depress nervous irritability. If the oil is not available, crush a teaspoon of the seeds and add that to just-boiled water. Steep, strain the liquid, and drink as tea.

Chamomile Drink chamomile during the day and before bedtime to dispel fatigue and nervousness. The tea may be used for infants.

Clove Add bruised cloves to any tea to relieve nervous irritability.

Lavender Add several drops of lavender oil to a pint of brandy. Use the liquid directly on the head for headaches. Lavender lotion or lavender water may also be used; there is an excellent English brand available at Caswell-Massey.

Lime or Linden Flowers Linden flower tea quiets the nerves and promotes sleep. The tea may also be used for infants.

Rosemary Rosemary relieves nervous palpitations of the heart, alleviates hysterical depressions, and lifts the spirits.

Valerian Valerian root has a strong smell; thus, the pills prepared from this valuable nerve-easing plant are usually small. A discote of valerian *on occasion* will relieve extreme nervous attacks, unease, nervous headache due to flatulence, or quiet the body after an unusual shock or excitement. Use this effective but strong pill, or expressed juice, or drops of tincture in water in moderation. Overuse is not advised.

NIPPLES

Carrot   Apply raw, scraped carrots directly to raw nipples.

Comfrey   Ointment of comfrey or fresh poultices of comfrey root or leaf will heal almost any body sore, including chapped or raw nipples. In many parts of Europe, especially France, nurses once applied the hollow part of the root directly over the sore or abscessed nipple.

Yarrow   Apply yarrow tea or expressed fresh yarrow juice compress to sore nipples.

NURSING

TO PROMOTE MILK FLOW

Borage   Drink a tea of borage leaves to increase the store of milk.

Dill   To avoid problems with excessive wind, feed infants mild dill tea. Prepare this by bruising a teaspoon of the seeds and steeping them in half a cup of boiling water; then strain the liquid.

Caraway   Caraway oil or tea will promote the secretion of milk. Add a few drops of the essential oil to any herbal drink, or make it as above.

Fennel   The Greeks use the entire plant as food and tea to encourage a milk flow in nursing mothers.

Fenugreek   Drink unstrained fenugreek tea during pregnancy and to increase breast milk.

Parsley Bruise the leaves, then apply them to hardened or knotty breasts and swollen glands during the nursing period, or apply a cloth that has been dipped into strong parsley tea.

Woodruff Infuse a handful of woodruff in wine for several days. Use up to 2 tablespoons of this liquid three times a day before meals to increase milk flow.

TO STOP MILK FLOW

Sage drink strong sage tea to dry up the milk flow during the weaning process.

PAIN RELIEF
(See also Liniment, Joints.)

Catnip Prepare a tea from sprays and flowers of the catnip plant. Use a very small amount in the morning or evening, or a teaspoon immediately before meals. Catnip tea soothes the nerves.

POISON IVY

Aloe Vera Apply plant juice from the inside of the leaf of this houseplant directly on poison-ivy blisters.

Goldenseal Make a thick paste or lotion from the powdered root, and apply it with, or without, apple cider vinegar. This helps to contain the spread of the poison on the skin and to relieve the itching.

Jewelweed This lovely yellow flower will frequently grow quite near poison ivy stands. Apply the sap from the stems for relief of itching. The potency of the plant varies from month to month.

Oatmeal   Add Aveeno, the colloidal oatmeal, to bathwater, and also use it as a paste on the poison ivy. Regular oatmeal may be blended into little particles and used in somewhat the same fashion.

Vinegar   Apple cider vinegar washes, splashes, and baths will relieve the itching.

Miscellaneous   Vitamin C (up to 3,000 milligrams) and tablets of pantothenic acid will help also to reduce the swelling. ash skin with brown soap and water and change clothing as soon as there is a known exposure.

POISONOUS PLANTS
(See Resources.)

POSTOPERATIVE TREATMENT

There are many vitamins that help recovery after an operation. I also believe strongly in the value of mobilizing one's internal energy and antibodies with directed medication on the area that has been operated on. This technique is so successful that it is now being used in certain cases to heal postoperative cancer sites.

Barley Broth   Barley broth is quite restorative and tasty. Simmer 1 cup of barley in 6 cups of water. Bring the water to a boil for two minutes. Let it stand for fifteen minutes. Strain out the barley and set it aside. Drink the water for strength during convalescence. The barley can also be eaten if the patient is hungry. If desired, the barley may be blended with honey to give it a pudding taste.

Castor Oil   Apply warm-to-hot castor oil over an incision *after* the stitches are removed. Castor oil will help prevent scarring.

RHEUMATIC PAINS

To eliminate uric acid crystals in the joints, drink parsley and/or juniper berry tea and lots of organic cranberry juice.

SINUS

Pack the area of pain with slightly wet, bruised peppermint leaves, or use a compress dipped in strong peppermint tea. Wind it around the bridge of the nose and the head.

SLEEP

Linden, chamomile, sage, catnip, clove, skullcap teas are all sedative. These can be mixed together according to personal choice and aroma, or may be used separately with, or without, some honey. Since honey absorbs water, it can be useful in holding moisture within the body, and can thus overcome the need for frequent bathroom visits during the night.

Wormwood, lavender, balm, chamomile compresses on the head will often help a nervous person to sleep better. ★

SMOKING—BREAKING THE HABIT

Chamomile ★   Chew chamomile flowers.

Gentian Root   Chew gentian root.

Miscellaneous ★   Take lots of saunas and steam baths to detoxify the body. Also drink large quantities of water to eliminate nicotine from the blood stream.

SNAKE BITE

Rue   While this in no way replaces a physician's attention to the bite, we use ice and bruised rue in cold beer on the bite, and drink the beer, too. Rue has an ability to expel poisons from the system.

SORES
(See also Bleeding, Boils, Bruises.)

Goldenseal and myrrh may be made into a paste with comfrey to heal almost any sore. Lemon will sometimes heal old sores. Honey will help to heal sores.

SPRAINS

Burdock   Drink burdock tea or apply burdock leaves as poultice.

Dock (Yellow)   Apply compresses of dock tea.

Ginger   Add ginger tea to bathwater, and soak in warm water.

Onion   Apply roasted onions, or cut up raw onions to apply to sprain in form of poultice.

Vinegar   Apple cider vinegar compresses often relieve the sprain.

SWEATING HERBS
(See Detoxify.)

It is very important to eliminate toxic materials through the pores of the skin. Various herbs have superior perspiration-inducing (diaphoretic) abilities. The most important of the diaphoretic herbs is yarrow. I use a combination of peppermint (over ½) and yarrow and elderblossoms at the onset of a cold or flu to induce sweating and settle the body. Other valuable sweat-inducing herbs are: chamomile, boneset, thyme, hyssop, and catnip—among many others.

SWELLING
(See also Inflammation.)

In addition to comfrey, plantain, apple cider vinegar, and witch hazel—which are explained under *Inflammation*—carrot poultice, castor oil packs, lavender lotion or lavender water, and bruised parsley poultice or parsley tea can be used to reduce swelling. While witch hazel is outstanding, some of the other herbs may be more healing.

THROAT
(See also Colds, Flu, Detoxification.)

Sage   Drink sage tea for a sore throat, and inhale sage-infused steam (add tea to the vaporizer). Sage will help open nasal and head passages.

Vinegar   Apply an apple cider vinegar compress to the throat, and bind it with a larger wool compress. This relieves even the most painful sore throat. Another useful combination is apple cider vinegar, wintergreen oil, and a tiny bit of cayenne pepper. Prepare ½ cup of apple cider vinegar. Add a teaspoon of wintergreen oil and a pinch of cayenne pepper. Soak strips of a brown paper bag (in case no cloths are available) in this preparation. Place the folded bag strip or wet cloth around the neck. Apply another dry wool cloth or, if that is not available, a large, double strip of brown paper or plastic to keep out the air.

TONIC HERBS

Alfalfa   Alfalfa is rich in vitamins and minerals. It will cleanse the whole system, and change it from acid to an alkaline state. This is useful, because most diseases develop concurrently with an excess acid state. Use alfalfa as a tea with honey and lemon or orange peel (dry your own organic lemon rind), or grow sprouts in your kitchen. Tablets are available.

Angelica   Use the stalk, making it into a cordial tea with honey. Angelica is good for the digestive system. Angelica candy is a tonic for the system.

Anise   Anise is a powerful tonic. Use bruised seeds for tea, or use anisette liqueur in small amounts, as if it were an anise tincture.

Basil   Basil tea is an excellent and important tonic for the system.

Carrot   Carrot juice is a tonic for the system.

Cayenne Pepper   Add a few grains of cayenne to any herbal tea to achieve a mild tonic effect.

Centaury   The whole plant is a bitter and useful tonic tea.

Peppermint   Peppermint leaves stimulate and warm the body and are excellent for the digestive and nervous systems. Note:

While this tea is readily available as a delicious and fragrant table tea, it should be alternated with other table teas.

Raspberry Raspberry leaves contain a substance which is very useful for all female organs. The leaves are a valuable tonic tea during pregnancy.

Watercress Watercress leaves are tonic. Eat some as often as possible.

URINATION PROBLEMS
(See Diuretic.)

VAGINITIS
(See also Suppositories.)

Acidophilus Prepare a douche with a capsule of acidophilus; use a capsule plus water in the douche. Acidophilus is a special culture usually made from goat's milk. The culture will enhance and replace missing intestinal and vaginal flora. This is useful after antibiotic treatment and to control the effects of a yeast infection.

Apple Cider Vinegar Add ½ to a whole cup to pint of warm water for an internal douche to control *Trichomonas vaginitis*. This acid medium is not suitable for a yeast infection. In both yeast and *trichomonas* infections you may use acidophilus and/ or a high-culture yogurt. If you are not sure what is causing the discharge and itching, check with your physician.

Yogurt Because it is cheaper and has a purer bacillus, buy a yogurt starter culture and make your own yogurt. Eat yogurt every day, and douche with diluted yogurt. As with the acidophilus, the proper yogurt bacillus also helps to replace intestinal and vaginal flora destroyed by previous antibiotic therapy.

VARICOSE VEINS

Cayenne Pepper   Add a few grains of cayenne pepper to every drink during the day, and work in up to ⅛ of a teaspoon as a dietetic supplement.

Marigold (calendula)   Bathe in marigold petal tea, and apply a marigold petal poultice and/or compress to the veined area. Cover with wool or plastic to keep wet. Drink tea of marigold leaves.

Oak Bark   Oak bark is very astringent but also contains calcium. The strong, concentrated tea should be used for frequent compresses. Cover the area with wool or plastic to keep it wet. A consistent program with oak bark decoction has proved quite successful. It certainly reduces the pain considerably.

Tansy   Use hot applications of tansy tea on large and knotted varicose veins, and replace the applications when they become cool. Cover them with wool or plastic to keep them wet and hot.

Wood Sorrel   Apply fresh wood sorrel leaves to the area of extended veins. Hold it on with large cabbage leaves and an "ace" type bandage.

WARTS

Apple Juice   Pare the wart, and spread the juice of a *sour* apple on the wart. The cure may be accomplished by the magnesia in the salts within the apple. (That is why a few grains of epsom salts also seem to work on many warts.)

Cabbage   Apply the juice of the white cabbage for a wart cure.

Chickweed   Add the juice of this wayside weed to warts, and they will eventually fall off.

Dandelion   In Derbyshire, England, as well as other places throughout the country, the juice from the stalk of the dandelion is applied to warts.

Fig Juice   Fresh green figs secrete a milky acrid liquid which will destroy warts.

Houseleek (or Hens and Chickens)   This succulent rock-garden and rooftop plant has thick fleshy leaves which contain a large proportion of supermalate of calcium. The juice is said to cure warts. The juice is also cooling for hornet and bee stings as well as burns. This juice is also a treasured home cosmetic ingredient.

Pineapple   Soak a small piece of absorbent cotton in fresh pineapple juice, or attach a bruised, runny piece of fresh pineapple to the corn or wart. Constant contact with the enzymes in the pineapple will gradually dissolve a pared-down wart or corn.

Watercress   Squeeze watercress juice on the wart.

WHITLOW
(Infected inflammation on finger—also called felon)

Lemon   Soak the finger in the juice of half a lemon.

WORMS
(Vermifuge)

Many herbs expel worms from the system. The following food herbs can be ingested safely and with pleasure to overcome this problem.

Carrots   Raw carrot salad was once used to expel worms from children. Use it with large amounts of fresh garlic to scour the system.

Cayenne   Mexican-Americans utilize cayenne pepper to eliminate various worms. The cayenne can be rolled in cream cheese "pills."

Garlic   Garlic is one of the most effective of the body cleansers and can be used daily in salads. To try a worm cure, use garlic "perles"—dried garlic rolled into pills—garlic in salad, and, most especially, eat a garlic bud first thing in the morning.

Horseradish   Fresh horseradish can be effective against some worms.

Lemon   Lemon water made with fresh, unstrained, but pitted lemons is cleansing for the system and will help eliminate worms in children.

Pumpkin   Eat pumpkin seeds freely to help expel a tapeworm.

(Dog) Rose (Hips)   The woolly down of the hips helps to expel roundworms from the system.

Tansy   An old English remedy to expel almost any type of worm: Eat the tansy seeds.

Thyme Eat thyme sprigs freely, or dried thyme in a sand-wich, or in pill form, or drink ½ cup of thyme tea each morning and evening to attempt to cleanse the system of worms.

Wormwood This is an ancient remedy. Use a sprig for a mild tea. But wormwood should *not* be taken over too long a time. One safe way would be to add a sprig to one of the tonic wines, and use a little bit at a time.

Important

Please refer to the Special Notice to the Reader on page *xx* and the instructions on page 117.

TRIP INSURANCE

Travel Tips

Dehydration

Overcome flight dehydration by drinking one glass of pure water for every hour of the flight. Avoid alcohol during any long trip. Overcome mouth and nose dryness with slippery elm or honey-glycerine lozenges. When you get home, make sure to use a cool moist air humidifier. This will help to prevent respiratory infections due to dryness or irritation.

Fatigue

On long-distance flights I always carry a collapsible rubber neck pillow. It is an excellent sleep aid.

I drink lots of herbal tea instead of coffee. I always carry ginseng tea extract for flights and eating out. I also carry a small vial of pure ginseng powder. I add a small pinch of this powder to the cup of boiling hot water I take with breakfast. To this cup of boiling water or herbal tea, I also add a teaspoon of combined equal amounts of apple cider vinegar and dark honey. I carry the cider vinegar and honey combination in a plastic vitamin jar. I reserve one small, sealed jar for every week of the vacation. The dose is one to several teaspoons a day in hot boiling water or in pure bottled cold water.

Both ginseng and apple cider vinegar restore flagging energy and preserve the body's energy balance.

Overcoming Pollution and Flight Fatigue

In addition to my personal dose of minerals and vitamins, I take large amounts of vitamin C, vitamin E, calcium panga-mate, and organic garlic capsules. All these substances help to overcome the effects of smog, nitrogen dioxide, and ozone toxicity.

Vitamin C: Dr. Szent Giorgy and Dr. Linus Pauling, in the *Journal of Applied Physiology and Science,* suggest rather large doses of 4 to 8 grams a day for antipollution control as well as for prevention of ozone toxicity.

Dr. Michael Walczak, Editor-in-Chief of the *Journal of Applied Nutrition,* comments on the value of disulfide com-pounds in protecting us against ozone pollution and avoiding any possible nitrogen dioxide and smog pollution. This com-pound is readily available to the body through the use of organic garlic extract, as garlic is high in sulphur.

Dr. Walczak also highly recommends water-soluble succi-nate type of vitamin E in doses of 1000 to 3000 units to help with the body's oxygen requirements in fighting ozone tox-icity. He notes that calcium pangamate also "has the property of increasing oxygen levels in the tissues and can be useful for the lowered cabin levels of oxygen and to retard fatigue.

"Travel fatigue can be lowered 50 to 75%," says Dr. Walczak, if these supplements and minerals were used during flights. He particularly recommends these substances to airline crews and pilots, as well as frequent air travelers.

Diarrhea

Nothing is as debilitating as travel-induced bacterial or viral gastrointestinal attacks. My prime preventives are acid-ophilus capsules and organic garlic capsules. The acidophilus culture, made from pure, unpasteurized goat's milk, like a good yogurt culture, replaces and fortifies normal intestinal flora. It will help you to resist most viral and bacterial invasions and most certainly help shorten any attacks. The garlic capsules act almost like an antibiotic.

I always carry peppermint tea bags and chamomile tea bags. These teas help digestive disturbances and will alleviate spasms.

A few drops of pure peppermint oil (you can obtain the oil in a drugstore) in peppermint tea will also act to control internal spasms and diarrhea. Peppermint extract may also be used.

Linden tea will also calm the body and help control spasms.

In the case of severe, debilitating diarrhea, sit for a few minutes at a time in a few inches of *cold* water.

Constipation

Many travelers react to changing climate, different water, and different food with constipation. To offset this possibility take *Inner-Clean* or *Swiss Kriss* herbal laxative tablets with you on your trip. The action is gentle and cleansing, and nongriping.

Insomnia

Drink chamomile and/or linden tea instead of coffee or tea. Even the most difficult insomnia will respond to consistent use of chamomile or linden.

For emergencies, overexcitement, or extreme sleeplessness, take one small discote of valerian (herb).

Emergencies/Accident

I always carry a vial of Rescue remedy, the five-flower combination of the Dr. Edward Bach flower remedy group. Each one of the five flowers helps with one or another emotional reaction during a possible acute emergency.

Important

Please refer to the Special Notice to the Reader on page xx and the instructions on page 117.

SECTION THREE

HOW TO MAKE THE HERBAL MEDICINES

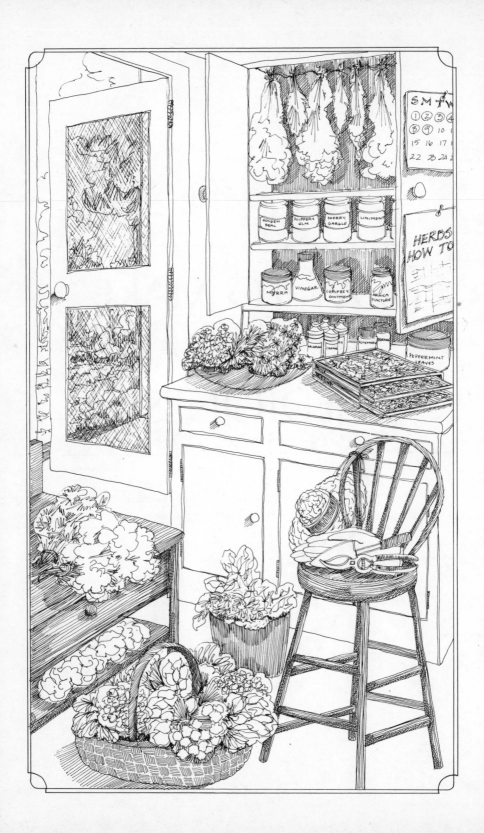

OBTAINING HERBS

You have many choices in your method of obtaining medicinal herbs. You can grow them in a garden or windowsill; pick them in the wild; purchase dried herbs from reliable botanical sources; buy food-herbs from markets; purchase tinctures, ointments, lotions, oils, liniments from botanical, homeopathic, or regular drugstores. There are many excellent mail-order sources listed in the *Resources* section.

Buying Dried Herbs

Seek out the best sources. Decide in what form you wish to purchase each plant. Leaves, flowers, resins, seeds, berries, and whole plants can come in *whole* form. Roots, rhizomes, resins, .leaves, flowers, stems, whole plants, and barks are available in *cut form*. This sometimes means small or large *chunks*, especially with roots. Seeds, bark, roots, buds, vegetables (such as red pepper), resins, berries, flowers, and leaves are available in *powdered* form.

You must specify the part you wish to purchase. For instance, in buying yarrow, the whole plant is usually sold, but I prefer to use the yarrow flowers. I never buy *cut* peppermint; it is usually a lot like peppermint dust. Therefore, I purchase only whole leaf peppermint. The same is true of chamomile flowers. Since these flowers are low growing, you risk getting ragweed in the dust if you buy powdered or cut chamomile, and that would increase the possibility of an allergic reaction.

Storage of Dried Herbs

All herbs must be stored to preserve their color and strength. I keep most of my fresh or dried herbs in strong, labeled, brown bags or in their paper container. I keep frequently used tea herbs in opaque containers on the food shelves in the kitchen. Others, I keep on a pantry shelf with a door. Because I usually have well over a hundred herbs available—many for demonstration or teaching purposes—I keep the bags, bottles, oils, tinctures, wines, liniments, gargles, brandies, and so on, in loose alphabetical order. Thus cocoa butter, calendula, comfrey, chamomile, and cayenne pepper are all in one grouping, and that makes them easier to find.

I keep first-aid oils, salves, and tinctures in the medicine chest. All medicinal herbs must be kept out of reach of children!

Dried herbs are potent for one year, but may often be used for as long as two years. See directions for making tinctures, extracts, oils, and other long-lived preparations.

Collecting Garden or Wild Herbs

While all parts of a plant contain chemicals, not all parts are valuable for teas or remedies. You will want to pick only the part or parts that will be of use to you. Therefore, you must learn which are the valuable medicinal parts. Furthermore, garden or wild herbs should be picked according to the nature of the part used. The plant will be more potent for home teas and preventive and remedial uses if gathered exactly when the special juices within the plant are most abundant.

Flowers Gather before or immediately after flowers open completely. Collect in clear, dry weather, in the morning after the dew has disappeared.

Leaves Gather leaves at full development just before the flower fades. Biennial leaves should be gathered during the second year when they are strongest. Collect in clear, dry weather, in the morning after the dew has disappeared.

Aromatic Herbs Gather when in flower. Collect leaves, flowers, or herbs in clear, dry weather, in the morning after the dew has disappeared.

Stalks Collect stalks in the autumn.

Twigs Collect twigs in the autumn.

Bulbs Gather bulbs after the new bulb is perfected, just before the leaves decay.

Barks Gather root, trunk, branch bark in either the fall or early spring. Separate and discard all decaying material. Use only the inner bark of slippery elm.

Seeds Collect seeds at the time of full maturity.

Rhizomes and Roots

Annuals:	Gather just before flowering.
Biennials:	Gather after vegetation of first year has ended.
Perennials:	Gather either in the spring before vegetation begins, or in the fall after vegetation ends.

DRYING AND STORING GARDEN OR WILD HERBS

Flowers Dry all flowers carefully and rapidly in order to preserve the color, as the strength of the flower can be judged by the intensity of its color. Take special care with flowers containing volatile oils.

Spread the flowers loosely on white paper. Do not dry scented flowers in the sun, for the sun depletes the strength of the plant. However, although aromatic flowers *must* be dried in the shade, they should be placed for a brief time in the sun, in order to prevent fungus attack.

Some flowers can be dried in medium-size bunches attached with string. Hang from a dowel or rafter in an airy room. For storage, hang bunches in a dry, airy room, or place in labeled brown paper bags. Fold bags to prevent insect attacks.

Leaves　Dry aromatic leaves in the shade. Place in the sun for a short time to prevent fungus attack. Unscented leaves may be dried in the sun, although it is best to dry them in an airy, dry place. Separate leaves, and change their position once they become dry. Succulent leaves need more care to prevent discoloration and may take more heat than dry, thin leaves.

Annual Plants and Tops　If the plants are not too juicy, they may be strung in bunches across the top of an airy, dry room.

Bulbs　Peel off the outer membranes, and cut the bulbs into transverse slices about a half inch in length. During the drying process they should be stirred and moved several times to prevent molding.

Barks, Woods, and Twigs　Dry in the sun or in thin layers in the open air. Do not dry wild cherry bark in the sun.

Fibrous Roots　Dry in the sun or artificially at temperatures from 65°F to 80°F.

Fleshy Roots and Rhizomes　Cut into transverse slices of about a half inch in length. Stir and move several times during the drying process to prevent attracting mold. Store in a cool, dry place.

Preserving Fresh Herbs By Freezing　I have been experimenting with an effective method of freezing fresh herbs. To my mind they taste even better than most dried herbs. Thus far I have frozen basil and parsley, but the method should work on a score of other window sill, garden or professionally grown herbs.

Wash each batch. Shake off the water. Spin dry them in a salad spinner. I find that my Swiss spinner really extracts all the water and the herbs seem even crisper. Next, place each batch in separate, closed plastic bags in the freezer. If you have a good freezer the herbs will be frozen within a few hours. Take the bags out of the freezer and break the herb fragments into tiny pieces. Insert these pieces into a clean, tight stoppered labeled jar. Keep it out of the sunlight.

SOME FIRST STEPS

Quality

Use only the best of substances. Buy only from reliable sources.

Advance Preparations

Have all cooking, storage, and labeling materials laid out in advance. This will prevent many last-minute crises. It is terribly disappointing to prepare an excellent but perishable syrup, and only then discover you don't have sterilized jars or paraffin sealer.

Decide in advance the preparation you intend to make, and make only one preparation at a time during a day or evening. Often an enthusiastic newcomer will attempt simultaneous preparation of ointments, syrups, and the like. By doing only one preparation at a time, you will remember precise procedures, and you won't feel anxious about timing and overlapping of various steps.

Quantity

If you collect your own garden plants or plants from the wild, gather together only the quantities you will be able to either dry or safely make ready as specific preparations. At times we have excitedly, almost greedily, collected large amounts of hawthorn haws or juniper berries, only to discover that we didn't have enough pots to make syrups or ointments or that we didn't have enough time to make the preparations after a long day in the wild.

So quantity depends on your facilities for cooking, your energy, your time, and proper storage materials.

Jars

Collect, wash, and sterilize jars of all sizes and shapes. Almost all of them will be useful at one time or another.

Ointments   You will need small jars with fairly wide openings for ointments. They will keep better. If you intend to keep the ointments for a long time, you will also need some sealing wax. Use either paraffin or beeswax.

You can often purchase small half- and one-ounce ointment jars from a friendly neighborhood pharmacist. They are a perfect size for gifts.

Tincture, Liniment, Gargles, Washes, Tonic Wines   All these preparations can be placed in any size jar. I find it most convenient to purchase small, inexpensive "flask" sizes of vodka, gin, brandy, or sherry. These are available in most urban centers but may have to be special-ordered by your liquor dealer. Since distilled spirits are the most effective liquid for long-time "storage" and since you may want to prepare only small batches of any one herb, the flask size is almost perfect. For instance, I just purchased several one hundred-proof Smirnoff vodkas in the 200 milliliter, 6.8 fluid ounce size for slightly over two dollars. Lower-proof brandies are slightly less expensive. Sometimes, it is convenient to also use the one-ounce bottles that are sold on airline flights. However, the lids are not always sturdy enough.

The directions for tonic wines, medicated wines, gargles, mouthwashes, washes, liniments, and tinctures will be found in this section.

HOW TO RELEASE HERBS FOR HOME REMEDIES

Locked Chemicals

The world contains hundreds of thousands of growing plants. While some are poisonous to eat or irritating to the touch (poison ivy, for instance), a surprising number of herbaceous plants, or other plant substances commonly called herbs, contain volatile oils, antibiotics, and aromatic or other healing chemicals. Some cultures, such as the Chinese, have thousands of plants in their *materia medica*. Other tribes, communities, or families know hundreds of such healing plants. But if we combine all groups, there are several thousand "good" plants that have been discovered over eons of time, through trial and error.

While occasionally a whole plant with stem, twig, flower, leaf, and bud is used for special preventive or remedial effect, usually only one part of a plant is used at a time. The whole plant or its various parts—such as berries, root, bark, resin, rhizome, stems, twigs, seeds, leaves, or flowers—can be considered a locked box of chemicals. If you want to use the chemicals within a plant, you must provide a specific key to unlock the box. This is true of both fresh and dried plant material. Incidentally, dried material is usually two to three times as strong as the fresh.

Releasing the Chemicals

The chemicals in plants may be released in a wide variety of ways. The method you use will depend on whether you are using fresh or dried material and whether you intend to use the material immediately or not. Other factors are the part of the body you wish to work on, whether the material is to be used externally or internally, as well as the remedial effect you wish to produce.

Plants react to stimuli. Some plants are soluble in water. Most leaves and flowers, some berries, and most pulverized or powdered materials are soluble in hot or standing cold water.

Most plant material will dissolve and can be extracted in a distilled alcohol medium. This is why I suggest the use of certain long-lasting wines and high-proof spirits. While rectified alcohol preserves the strained "extraction," you can also add a few drops of vegetable or animal glycerine, or drops of tincture of benzoin to further preserve any preparation.

Containers

Use glass, ceramic, stainless steel, or smoothly glazed cast iron. Do not use Teflon or aluminum. Metals are sometimes corroded by the plant ingredients, so glass, glazed ceramic, or earthenware products are best choices. Do not use iron pots when astringent vegetables are being prepared for herbal remedies, but clean cast iron is preferred over any copper or brass pots, which must never be used in preparing herbs.

Methods

Herbs can be powdered or bruised and added to such solvents as boiling or cold water, milk, vinegar, rectified alcohol (gin, vodka, or brandy will do), wine, fat, or oil. Herbs can be roasted (for example, dandelion roots or chick peas) or used bruised or wet in the form of external poultices. Many herbs can be added to a variety of water baths—foot, arm, full body, and so on—to detoxify the body, relieve pain, release tension, relieve itching (oatmeal), soften the skin, or bring blood to the surface of the skin (mustard powder paste).

Herbs can be absorbed into fats or oils to produce softening, healing creams, ointments, or massage aids. They can be added to alcohol, vinegar, or water for body rubs; to water or sherry for delicious mouthwashes; or combined in dry form for tooth and mouth aids. Herbs can be added to various materials to produce excellent healing douches, colonic irrigations, insect repellents, healing syrups, lozenges, pills, deodorants, suppositories, and other specific health aids.

Important

Please refer to the Special Notice to the Reader on page xx and the instructions on page 117.

METHODS AT A GLANCE

Never Use Aluminum to Prepare Herbs

Water

Infusion
The most common form of everyday use for herbs is tea.

Hot Infusion
Pour boiling water over an herb. Steep for fifteen minutes. Strain. This method is usually used for leaves and flowers to make instant tea for drinking. Powdered bark, root, seeds, and resin and *bruised* nuts, seeds, bark, and buds are also receptive to steeping in boiling water.

Cold Infusion
Steep in cold water or cold milk for several hours.

Wet, mashed herbs can be used internally as a tea or as poultices on the body.

Waters
Steeped herbs, water, and alcohol and steeped herbs plus honey and other fruits are often called waters. Sometimes extracts or spirits of various herbs (lavender, for instance) are also called waters.

Decoction

This is the second most frequently used method of extracting chemicals.

Hard parts of plants, such as twigs, roots, barks, rhizomes, berries, and some seeds, only release volatile oils and locked-in chemicals when they are gently *simmered* for about thirty minutes in water. Strain and use.

Long simmering will produce a distillation, or extract, of an herb. This is similar to a soup.

Alcohol

Tincture

Herbs not soluble in water are usually soluble in rectified alcohol or spirits. A tincture is a solution of a medicinal substance in alcohol or diluted alcohol. Coarse, bruised, or pulverized material is usually used. The material is placed directly in the bottle, or alcohol may be *filtered* through the plant material. To filter, use coffee parchment cones.

Medicated wines are tinctures of a less stable nature.

Oils

Aromatic oils and rectified alcohol can be combined. The oils seep into the alcohol to produce an essence. See *Oils.*

Vinegar

Tincture

Herbs that are soluble in alcohol are frequently soluble in vinegar, and such steeping of fresh or dried plant materials is useful for salad vinegars, cosmetic vinegars, some liniments, and preventive, sickroom "washes."

Fat

Ointments

Fresh or dried herbs, herb oils, or herb tinctures and

extracts heated together with any variety of fats produce healing salves. Add wax for hardness.

Cold Cream
Mix lanolin (fat), oil, rosewater, and wax.

Suppository
Heat a fat, herb, and wax, or preferably cocoa butter and healing herb for cylinder shaping and insertion in rectum or vagina.

Lip Balm
Combine oils, honey, beeswax, vanilla.

Oils

Essence
Oils may be "captured" by evaporation from flower petals. Also, vegetable, nut, or fruit oils can be used as a medium for steeping aromatic plants to extract volatile oils. Aromatic oils can also be steeped in alcohol to extract essence.

Combinations
Combine oils for healing, massage, insect repellent, or lip balm.

Juice

Essence or Extract
Extract a juice of a plant by applying pressure.

Sugar

Alcohol and sugar have many similar chemical components, and sugar will preserve many plant materials.

Syrup
Combine sugar, water, and plant, or sugar, water, plant, and spirits.

Jelly
Syrup in more congealed form.

Electuary
Use powder to make a syrup.

Conserve
Beat together sugar and plant material.

Lozenge
Pill made of solid plant material, sugar, and gummy material.

Dried Material

Pills
Roll bruised or pulverized plant material into pellets, place in glycerine capsules, or work with sugar into cake-like lozenges. Combine dried material for various insect repellents, potpourri, rodent repellent, herb deodorant, and herb salts.

Combinations
Single-herb or combinations of herbs may be steeped to make a drinking tea, a decoction, or, steeped in alcohol, vinegar. Steeped, strained material may be used for douching and rectal irrigation purposes.

Laxative
Single-herb or combinations of herbs can be used for laxative purposes.

Breath Sweeteners
Eat breath-sweetening seeds such as caraway, fennel, or anise, or steep these and other seeds and spices in sherry to make breath-sweetening gargles and mouthwashes.

Liniment
Add dried herbs to vinegar, oils, alcohol, or water to produce friction rub.

Tooth Preparations
Combine dried herbs and other materials for tooth aids.

THE METHODS

INFUSION

Leaves and flowers and some whole plants are soluble in liquids, usually water. There are two kinds of infusions: hot and cold.

The cold infusion consists of a soaking in cold water or milk for several hours. The herb is then strained. Use a cold infusion when the active principles of the plant are highly volatile or when it could be injured by heat. This will be noted in the text. Occasionally milk infusions are used to increase the healing ability of herb poultices and compresses.

The hot infusion—the most frequently used of all herb preparations—is produced by pouring boiling water over the herb or herb part and steeping the infusion in a covered container for fifteen minutes to a half hour, or even longer if the infusion is to be used cold. Herbal "teas" are usually infusions. Some are decoctions (see below).

To Make an Infusion

Usually 1 teaspoon of an herb to 1 cup boiling water is sufficient. But you may use more for weak teas. Use 2 teaspoons of a fresh herb. Leaves, flowers, and berries should be slightly bruised to help release their aromatic oils.

When making aromatic teas for table use, warm the teapot slightly, steep the herb for a few minutes, and then strain the liquid into your cup. Herbal teas may be used piping hot with bruised seeds such as fennel, anise, caraway, coriander, or cumin for both taste and stomach-easing qualities, or cold, or with ice. In the summer we make up big batches of peppermint tea and keep it in the refrigerator. But there are many excellent combinations of herbal blends you can make yourself.

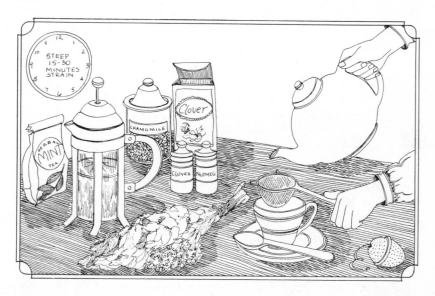

To Preserve an Infusion for Medicinal Use

1. Strain the infusion while hot, and pour it into a bottle with a tight stopper. The bottle must be quite filled, and the stopper made to displace its own bulk of liquid. The hotter the liquid and the freer it is from air bubbles, the better the infusion will keep. A bottle with a perforated cork stopper may also be used, and the hole instantly closed with a sealing wax.

2. Another way to preserve an infusion is to make a very concentrated tea, actually three times as strong as the ordinary infusion. Add 1 part alcohol to every 3 parts infusion. (With ¾ cup infusion, use ¼ cup alcohol.) Since this infusion will be three times as strong as the average infusion, it may be diluted with three measures of water and used when needed.

Medicinal Teas

One of my grandmother's frequent dictums concerning the suitability of an herb for a particular person and condition was: "If the tea smells bad and tastes bad, it isn't right; but if it smells quite pleasant and possibly tastes bad, it can be tried out."

But not all herbs are safe to ingest (or use on the body either). Indeed, some herbs are hazardous to your health. The best method of using herbs is to learn about them one at a time, and to use them one at a time. Read up on the herbs. Evaluate them carefully. Know the herbs you use!

Some herbs appear to have long and distinguished folk medicine use and to be non-toxic, and yet may still be listed as dangerous for some internal or external use by some government agency. On the other hand, many of the warnings may be appropriate and should be seriously investigated. Since there are so many safe and valuable herbs and food herbs, why take a chance with any herbs that may work negatively on the central nervous system, or other systems for that matter.

It is particularly important to use small (half or less) doses of herbs for children, and to experiment with possible allergic reactions to any herbs before using them in quantity.

Quantities/Time In using medicinal infusions or decoctions (see the next section after *Infusion*), especially for an acute health problem, drink only half a cup three times a day, preferably a half hour before each meal. When the symptoms of the health problems disappear, discontinue taking the tea. If no change is seen after three days, change the treatment, as three days is about what it takes for an herbal tea to work.

On the other hand, don't be discouraged if you feel "badly" after an hour or so or during the first day or so. Many herbs start to normalize the body, and detoxify and push out old wastes. This happens very often with ginger tea and in eating cinnamon sticks, both of which are extremely detoxifying. Give a tea a chance to work, but remember: Each person is different, and there is no one tea that works for everyone. You have to experiment.

Herbs for Home Table Teas

There are about twenty-five to fifty delicious herbs that may be used separately, or in a variety of combinations, according to your need, mood, and the season.

In the past, I mainly used peppermint as my everyday tea because of its stimulating aroma and pleasant taste. But because peppermint has a high amount of tannin, I now vary my selection of table teas a lot more. While I am traveling, though, I never fail to take tea bags of both peppermint and chamomile, since both these teas have a benign influence on digestion. I also carry a small vial of either peppermint oil or peppermint extract. Either one of these concentrated peppermints may be used, a few drops at a time, in a cup of boiled, hot water.

Other teas that I like are linden flowers (lime flowers), alfalfa leaves and alfalfa seeds, chamomile flowers, red raspberry leaves, yarrow flowers, elderflowers, clover flowers (when I collect them myself, I use the stems and all), desert herb tea, and hawthorn berry tea.

Here are some of the everyday herbs that I either grow, pick in the wild, or purchase in dry form:

Flowers Chamomile, elderflower, clover, linden, yarrow, mullein.

Leaves, Peppermint, spearmint, pennyroyal, alfalfa, bee balm, blackberry, blueberry, catnip, costmary, horsetail, hyssop, lemon balm, oatstraw, parsley, red raspberry, rosemary, sage, thyme.

Berries Blueberry, hawthorn, juniper, raspberry, rose hips.

Seeds Anise, alfalfa, caraway, celery, coriander, cumin, dill, fennel, fenugreek.

Bark   Cherry, cinnamon.

Root   Comfrey, ginger, ginseng.

Stem   Desert or Mormon tea, clover flowers and stems.

Rind   Organic rind from peeled oranges, lemons, grapefruit—
especially orange.

Favorite Herb Tea Blends

Combine in advance and place in labeled jars or paper
bags:

Peppermint-Alfalfa Tea Blend [Purifier]

> 1   cup peppermint or spearmint or bee balm
>   leaves
> 1   cup dried alfalfa leaves

Lemon Mint Blend [Digestive aid, cold aid]

> ½   cup dried peppermint leaves
> 1   cup dried alfalfa leaves
> 3   tablespoons dried lemon balm leaves
> 3   tablespoons dried, grated organic lemon
>   rind

Hot Mint Tea [Cold aid, digestive aid]

> 1   peppermint tea bag
> 1–2 teaspoons crème de menthe liqueur
> 1   cup boiling water

Pour boiling water over the teabag. Steep for three
minutes or slightly longer. Add the liqueur. A wonderful drink
on a cold night. Excellent for colds and digestive problems.

Rose Hip Tea Blend [Vitamin C drink]

1   cup dried rose hips
1   3-inch stick cinnamon
¼   cup dried lemon balm leaves
1   teaspoon dried, grated organic lemon
    rind

Rose Hip and Blackberry Cordial [Restorative]

2   teabags rose hips (Pompadour brand)
1–2 teaspoons blackberry cordial
1   cup boiling water

Steep together and serve.

Ginger-Strawberry Tea Blend [Anticold, stimulant]

1   teaspoon ginger powder
1   cup of any dried mint leaves
2   cups dried strawberry leaves

Clover Tea [Body-cleanser]

20 clover blossoms, stems and all
4   Queen Anne's lace seedheads—pick
    when they are starting to turn brown-
    black
1   cup boiling water

Add boiling water and steep for five minutes.

Clover Tea Blend [Detoxifier]

2   cups clover blossoms
2   thin sticks cinnamon, slightly bruised
1   teaspoon grated, dried organic orange
    rind

Caraway Julep for Infants [Digestive aid]

>1–2 teaspoons caraway seeds
>1   cup cold water

Bruise seeds and stand in the cold water for six hours (cold infusion). Strain. Give infant 1–3 teaspoons a day, 1 teaspoon at a time. This helps with digestive problems.

Fennel [Thirst quencher]

>1½ quarts fennel seed tea
>1   large, 46-ounce can unsweetened pineapple juice
>1   quart apple cider or orange juice

Combine all ingredients and chill. Serve very cold. Yield: 1 gallon.

Herbal Breakfast Drink

>1   quart chamomile tea (Rose hips may be substituted)
>1   large, 46-ounce can pineapple juice
>2   ripe bananas
>2   cups yogurt (or kephir)
>1   quart orange juice
>Juice of 4 fresh limes

Make tea and strain. Combine with pineapple juice. Blend bananas and yogurt together until smooth. Add chamomile, orange juice, and lime juice. Serve very cold.

This makes up into a gallon for a large crowd.

Elderberry Flower Tea Blend

>1   cup dried elderflowers
>2   teaspoons anise seed
>1   cup dried alfalfa
>1   teaspoon grated, dried organic orange rind

Ginger Ale [Digestive aid]

    1   large piece ginger root, bruised
    1   pint boiling water
    1   tablespoon honey
        Perrier water as needed

Boil water, add bruised ginger root, and simmer for fifteen to twenty minutes. Strain out root. Add honey and mix well. Combine with Perrier water. Don't use powdered ginger.

Weed Juice and Pineapple [Vitamin-rich]

        Mint
        Alfalfa
        Filaree
        Dandelion
        Romaine leaves
        Parsley
        Celery tops
        Carrot tops
    2   cups pineapple

Combine handfuls and extract into juice.

Place handfuls of these weeds and home greens in the juice extractor, and use 1 cup to each 2 cups of pineapple. This green juice may be made into ice cubes and used.

Mint-Strawberry Ice Cubes   Combine a bruised mint leaf and half a strawberry, add to each ice cube section. Use in summer drinks.

Chamomile Summer Punch [Tonic]   Chamomile flowers are mild, digestive, and tonic. A strong infusion with pineapple, papaya, and honey provides a delightful summer punch. Add mint and strawberry ice cubes for color and taste. If you are using a large punch bowl, freeze ice in a small decorative mold or refrigerator storage container, since large cakes dissolve slowly.

> 1   gallon pineapple juice (chilled in advance)
> 1   pint papaya juice (concentrate) (chilled in advance)
> 4–5 handfuls chamomile
>   Several teaspoons honey
> 1   gallon boiling water
>   Ice cubes or ice mold

Boil water, and steep chamomile flowers for ten minutes. Strain out. Cool. Refrigerate. Combine with pineapple juice, papaya concentrate, and honey. If necessary, combine half at a time. Be certain your chamomile flowers do not include stray ragweed.

Winter Punch (for 4 persons) [Body balancer]

> 4   tart apples
> 2   lemons
> 5   cups water
> 4   tablespoons honey
> 4   tablespoons apple brandy (or cider)

Wash and quarter the apples and lemons. Place in glass or enamel pot, add water, and bring to a boil. Lower the heat immediately, and simmer for about ten minutes. Warm large teapot, and strain into teapot. Place 1 teaspoon honey and 1 teaspoon cider or brandy in each of four cups, and add the hot apple-lemon nectar.

Hot Roasted Chickpea Tea

Roast dried chick peas in the oven until they turn a dark brown. Grind them in a nut or coffee grinder.

> 1   cup boiling water, plus several table-spoons to offset evaporation
> 1   teaspoon chickpea grinds

Simmer the grinds and water together for seven minutes. Strain and drink piping hot. This tastes a lot better than dandelion or chicory root coffee and has more nutrition and none of the acid side effects of real coffee.

WATERS

Rosemary Water

4   tablespoons rosemary flowers
1   nutmeg, grated
2   tablespoons cinnamon, grated
1   quart alcohol spirit

Stand and steep for ten days. Strain.

Barley Waters

Both barley waters are used to aid invalids, to add nutrition to people who find it hard to eat, and to alleviate diarrhea, especially in infants.

Simple Barley Water

4   ounces barley, whole
2   ounces honey
    Lemon peel, washed
½   lemon

Add 1 pint of water to barley and lemon peel. Simmer until soft. Remove from heat. Steep. Add honey.

Compound Barley Water

2   pints simple barley water
1   pint hot water
2½   ounces sliced figs
½   ounce, sliced and bruised licorice root
2½   ounces raisins

Boil down to 2 pints. Strain.

DECOCTIONS

When a plant is not soluble in standing cold or boiling hot water, it will often yield its soluble ingredients by simmering in almost boiling water for 30 minutes or more. This simmering of roots, barks, resins, rhizomes, and berries is called decoction. In effect, you are making a soup stock from a tough plant substance.

For decoctions, fresh herbs should be sliced; dry herbs should either be powdered or well bruised.

Decoctions should always be strained while hot, so that the matter which separates on cooling may be mixed again with the fluid by shaking when the remedy is used.

Use glass, ceramic, or earthenware pots, or clean, unbroken enameled cast iron. Do not use plain cast iron with astringent plants.

Examples of plants to be decocted: elm bark, uva ursi, barley, flaxseed, broom, quince seed, comfrey root, cherry bark, oak bark, and some gum resins. You may preserve decoctions in the same way you preserve infusions.

TINCTURES

In the medicinal sense, tinctures are solutions of medicinal substances in alcohol or diluted alcohol. Apple cider vinegar may be used for some special preparations. These are explained in the *Vinegar* section.

Tinctures in alcohol are prepared by steeping herbs in the rectified spirits or alcohol, by heating herbs and alcohol at various temperatures, or by filtering alcohol through herbs suspended in a parchment cone filter. This last is accomplished in the same way coffee is made in some coffee makers, except that soluble plant material drips down through the filter and the herb-impregnated alcohol is then used.

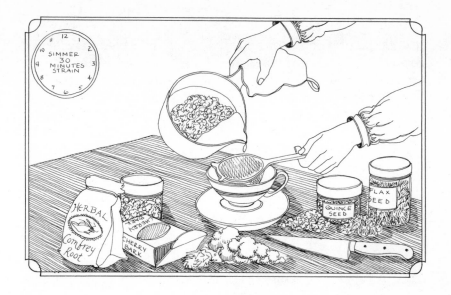

Alcohol

This alcohol is not rubbing alcohol, but rather ninety-proof spirit or, if the tincture is to be used internally, a ninety-proof vodka or gin. I also often use an eighty- or eighty-six-proof brandy or whiskey for tinctures, and I have found them quite acceptable. I often use herbs steeped in sherry for mouthwashes and gargles. I frequently use vinegar tinctures as body washes, liniments, and for healing compresses.

Dosage

An alcohol solution dissolves all the chemical principles of a plant and acts to preserve it for further use. Since tinctures are very concentrated extracts of herbs preserved in alcohol, very little is needed. Use from five to an average of fifteen drops at a time.

A drop of tincture is equal to a teaspoon of the herb juice.

When to Use

Use drops of the tincture added to hot or cold herb teas for additional preventive or remedial action, or added to water for external use in compresses, foot baths, and arm baths.

Add drops of healing tinctures to oils or fats to create an instant healing ointment, to cocoa butter for healing or special-acting suppositories, or to dried herbs for pills or lozenges.

Basic Tincture Technique

The easiest home preparation is made by steeping herbs in either vodka, gin, whiskey, or brandy. This way I always know that my tinctures can be used internally when necessary.

> 1   pint ninety-proof* vodka or gin
> 1–4 ounces cut form of herb, depending on the strength of the herb (4 ounces are best)

Steep the cut herb (powders tend to get stringy) for two weeks. Strain out the herb or herbs. Label the bottle.

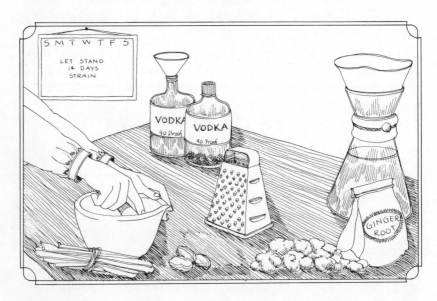

*Whiskey or brandy, eighty- to eighty-six-proof, may also be used for short-term tinctures.

For a Stronger Tincture

Filtering ninety-proof alcohol through coarse herbs can produce a strong tincture. Place the herbs in a cone-shaped parchment. Pass the filtered alcohol repeatedly through the powdered or cut herb. Catch the slow drippings in a jar or the bottom of a clean glass coffeemaker. When it has passed once, you may use it, but the more you repeat the process, the stronger the tincture will be. Label the jar.

Adding Water

It is possible to dilute any alcohol tincture. This is an acceptable pharmaceutical technique.

If you wish to extend the amount of tincture, add 4 ounces of water and 1 teaspoon of glycerine for every pint of alcohol. The glycerine is optional, but additional preservative is often used by professional pharmacists.

Some Tinctures

Compound Tincture of Lavender   This recipe is given to show how several oils and powders may be combined. This tincture is prepared by filtration. It is a lovely compound of spices and can be used along with other herbal medicines. It is an old remedy for gastric uneasiness, nausea, and flatulence.

The dose is 7 drops on ¼ lump of sugar, 15 drops on ½ a lump, 30 drops on a whole lump. Or the sugar may be mixed with several tablespoons of water, and the drops added to the water.

> ¼   fluid ounce oil of lavender
> ¼   fluid ounce oil of rosemary
> ½   ounce cinnamon powder
> ¼   ounce fine nutmeg powder

1   handful moderately fine red saunders
     powder
1½ pints alcohol
2   cups water

Dissolve the oils in the alcohol. Add the water. Mix the powders. Moisten the mixture with a fluid ounce of the alcoholic solution of the oils. Pack it into a conical percolator such as the Chemex, and gradually pour over it the remainder of the alcoholic solution.

Calcium Tincture for Daily Calcium Needs [Vinegar tincture]
★   Break open a dozen eggs. Place the yolks and eggs aside for food use. Dry the eggshells, and pull out the membranes. Blend dried egg shells into powder in a blender or mortar. Add to a pint of apple cider vinegar, but use a quart to a 2-quart bottle, as the preparation creates a lot of fizzle. Put on bottle cap immediately. Use 1 tablespoon three times a day.

We also use this old-fashioned folk-medicine tincture combined with honey, as the apple cider vinegar and honey combination provides needed hydrochloric acid. If deficient, use more—2 tablespoons three times a day. Do not use if ulcers are present.

Keep refrigerated.

Ice Lemon Vodka Drink

1   fifth or quart bottle minus ¼ cup vodka
3   lemons
1–2 teaspoons sugar
¼   teaspoon salt
5   drops glycerine

Remove large pieces of washed rind from the lemons, and place the pieces into the bottle. Add the sugar, salt, and glycerine. Seal, and refrigerate. Before serving, place the bottle in the freezer for three hours.

Essence

See later references to oils steeped in alcohol to produce aromatic essence.

MEDICATED WINES

Technically, anything steeped in an alcoholic medium will be a tincture, but wine has less alcohol than the ninety-proof spirits called for in pharmaceutical tinctures. Most wines are categorized by the percentage of alcohol they contain. Double the percentage to find the proof. So the highest proof in wine would be about thirty-proof. Light-colored wines, usually the lowest in alcohol content, tend to decompose rather quickly, as compared to the tinctures, which will last for as long as you will ever need them.

However, wine is rather inexpensive and has some long-range advantages in plant medicine. Because of its alcohol content (even though lower than that of vodka, gin, and brandy), it immediately dissolves any plant substances which are normally insoluble in water. Alcohol helps to resist the tendency to spontaneous change in all plants, and the grape acid also helps to increase the solvent power of the wine.

Wine is also less stimulating for the body than the high-proof spirits and can be used for sipping in small quantities, while the tinctures may only be used by the teaspoon.

Not any wine will do. Use a full-bodied red wine for tonic wines. In my experience, Madeira holds up well, tastes wonderful, and is just the right base for a tonic.

I use inexpensive sherries for the mouthwashes and gargles, and although light wines tend to decompose easily, I find they hold up quite well with the addition of the herbs. See *Breath Sweeteners.*

Make all these medicated wines in small quantities and *without* heat. Keep the wines well-corked and in a cool place.

Some Medicated Wines

My Favorite Tonic Wine ★   Sip this wine any time you feel ill, or use after meals (a tablespoon at a time) as a tonic wine. This wine is marvelous when you feel run down or if you can't eat anything because of a flu or other illness. Some students have confided that this wine has tided them over during difficult illnesses.

> 1 pint Madeira
> 1 sprig wormwood
> 1 sprig rosemary
> 1 small bruised nutmeg
> 1 inch bruised ginger root
> 1 inch bruised cinnamon bark
> 12 large organic raisins

Pour off about an ounce of the wine. Place herbs in the wine. Cork the bottle tightly. Place the bottle in a dark, cool place for a week or two. Strain off the herbs. Combine this medicated wine with a fresh bottle of Madeira. Mix thoroughly. Sip a small amount at a time whenever needed. I often use the undiluted wine. It helps to settle the stomach, gives energy, and, well, just makes you feel better.

Wormwood Wine [To settle the stomach and offset the ill effect of alcohol]   Wormwood is a bitter herb. The Romans used it before and after an alcohol binge to counteract the effects of drinking too much alcohol. Gentian is another bitter digestive aid that will quickly settle an upset stomach. One of the bitter tastes of Campari, the marvelous Italian aperitif (before-dinner drink), comes from wormwood. Campari can be used in teaspoon amounts to settle the stomach. Otherwise, add a sprig of wormwood to any leftover white wine, and steep for one to two weeks. Do not ever use much in any preparation.

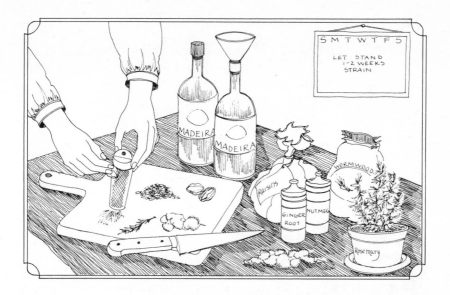

Chamomile Wine [To settle the stomach]

1 bottle white wine or Maderia red wine
1 handful chamomile flowers

Add the flowers to the wine. Steep for a week to ten days. Strain. Use in tablespoon doses to settle the stomach. Chamomile flowers help to alleviate body spasms and colic. Dip a folded cloth in the wine and place the compress on abdominal area.

Rosemary Wine [A sedative cordial] ★

1 bottle white wine
1 handful fresh rosemary leaves or 2 tablespoons dried leaves
2 tablespoons dried borage leaves

Steep leaves in white wine for about a week or so. Strain out the herbs. Use in small quantities whenever needed. This wine can lift the spirits from a mild depression, and it also quiets the nerves.

Aromatic Wine [Tonic, digestive aid] This French formula

possesses strong tonic and aromatic properties. It is useful for invalids with feeble digestions and will also help with flatulence and other digestive disturbances.

2   pints claret (Bordeaux) wine
2   tablespoons sage leaves
2   tablespoons thyme leaves
2   tablespoons hyssop leaves
2   tablespoons spearmint leaves
2   tablespoons wormwood leaves
2   tablespoons marjoram herb

Chop the herbs into a coarse powder. Moisten the powders with some of the claret. Pack into a Chemex coffee machine, using parchment paper. Pour the claret over the herbs. It should yield about 1 pint of filtered liquid.

Use 1 tablespoon at a time. For ulcers, use heated as a hot (external) *compress* (dip a cloth into the hot liquid).

Antichill, Anticold Ginger Wine [or whiskey] ★

1   pint brandy
    Several pieces fresh bruised ginger root

Steep 1–2 tablespoons of bruised ginger root in an inexpensive bottle of brandy (or whiskey) for a week to ten days. Strain out. Use in teaspoon doses when you have a cold or chill, or add a teaspoon to hot peppermint or sage tea. Ginger will not only detoxify the body, but also will induce perspiration. This helps to combat a cold.

VINEGAR

Vinegars have many medical uses. You can make your own apple cider vinegar or blackberry vinegar, or you can add certain medicinal or culinary herbs to commercially prepared vinegars.

Apple cider vinegar is one of my favorite external and internal medicines. To make a restorative, refreshing, energizing drink which also helps to dissolve arthritic and gouty deposits, combine a tablespoon of uncooked honey and a tablespoon of a good apple cider vinegar. Add to a glass of water. A little less honey may be used if you are making a pitcherful. This drink is good for small children (not newborn infants, though), as this ancient combination of sweet and sour plus water normalizes the body.

The apple cider vinegar is useful externally to alleviate pain and help reduce sprains. I use at least a cup at a time in the bath to alleviate muscle soreness. I also splash it directly on my shoulders, arms, chest, and torso to restore flagging energy. I don't really know why apple cider vinegar patted on the body or placed in the bathwater will overcome body fatigue, but it does.

Diluted apple cider vinegar may be used in small amounts to help reduce fever and may also be splashed or sponged on the patient to reduce the temperature. Sponge the body in sections and friction dry, and do not allow the rest of the body to be in a draft. Blackberry vinegar may also be used in the same way in relation to fever.

Herb vinegars—and here, especially, note the justifiably famous Vinegar of the Four Thieves—may be used to cleanse sickrooms and wash the body during any bacterial illness or during epidemics.

Making Vinegar at Home

You will need a wide-mouthed jar or crock, a cover for the crock, and the peelings, cores, and bruised apples left after making apple sauce or apple pie. Place the leftover pieces of apple in the crock, and cover with cold water. Place the top on the crock, and store it in a warm place. Occasionally lift the cover and add whatever additional peels, cores, and apple pieces you can. Strain off the froth as you go along. When the vinegar smells and tastes right, strain out the apple pieces. Pour the vinegar into sterilized bottles, and cork for further use. Label.

A Cider Vinegar Shortcut

Aeration is the answer to souring a vinegar. Also, if you wish to quicken the fermentation process, add a small amount of live yeast in a brown paper to your crock or keg.

To aerate as farmers once did, keep two barrels with spigots. In one barrel, make the vinegar as described above. In the second barrel, keep matchstick-thin sticks of birch or beech boards. After a few days, open the faucet and allow the cider to dribble through the birch or beech boards. As soon as the second barrel fills up, pour the vinegar into the first barrel again. This process may be repeated several times.

Some Vinegars

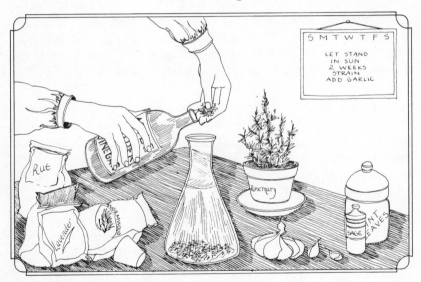

Blackberry Vinegar ★

    4   pounds fresh blackberries
          Enough malt vinegar to cover blackberries
    1   pound sugar for every pint extracted blackberry juice*

*Sugar can be replaced with glycerine. See the recipe for *Blackberry Glycerite*.

Wash the blackberries in cold running water. Place in a glass, earthenware, or ceramic pot. Cover with malt vinegar for three days. Stir once a day. Strain through a sieve, and drain thoroughly by placing a plate on top and putting a weight on the plate. Let it drip all day. Measure the juice, and allow 1 pound of sugar per pint of juice (for external use, glycerine is preferred—see next recipe). Simmer in another glass, ceramic, or earthenware pot for five minutes. Collect and discard the top scum. Cool, bottle, cork, and label.

This vinegar is excellent for fevers, arthritis, and gout. The dose here is 1 tablespoon dissolved in a large cup of distilled water. Use three times a day. This preparation will somewhat ease the pain and is said to eventually help dissolve arthritic deposits. This vinegar is also said to be good for anemia and may be used with advantage by many heart patients.

Blackberry Glycerite ★   The recipe for this is almost the same as that for blackberry vinegar, but glycerine is used instead of the sugar. For every pint of the extracted juice, use 8 ounces of glycerine (½ pint). Simmer the blackberry vinegar and glycerine together for five minutes. Skim. Cool and place in a sterilized, labeled bottle. Store in a cool place.

This glycerite of blackberry can be used in the same way as the vinegar. For painful joints, heat this preparation in small quantities, dip in a folded cloth. Several times a day apply hot cloths to painful joints.

Vinegar of the Four Thieves ★   This is one of the most interesting legends in the fascinating history of herbalism. There is a possibility that this remedy was used and devised by an apothecary, Richard Forthave, and that the success and usefulness of the remedy created its own myth. This recipe has been in use for centuries, but the legend has it that it was discovered during a devastating bubonic plague.

Four thieves who had safely ransacked empty plague-ridden houses were caught by policemen and brought before the French judges in Marseilles. The judges wondered aloud how these thieves had resisted the plague, especially since they were in and out of plague-infested homes.

"We drink and wash with this vinegar preparation every few hours," they answered.

In return for giving the recipe, the thieves were given their freedom.

There are several Four Thieves vinegars. I extracted the simplest recipe from the notebook of a Virginia housewife. She combined a handful of each of the antidisease herbs and steeped them in apple cider vinegar. After the initial two-week steeping (a vinegar tincture), she added garlic buds.

This aromatic and antibacterial vinegar is an excellent wash for floors, walls, sinks, bedsteads, pots, and pans, in sickrooms, bathrooms, and kitchens. It will offset a damp-weather smell in a house and be a helpful floor and wall wash in a room overcrowded with people.

Externally, this vinegar may be used in small proportions in a bath or diluted for body wash. Ordinary apple cider vinegars may be used in undiluted state if desired, but some of the herbs in this recipe are too strong for the skin, and the vinegar must be diluted.

Internally, the dose is a teaspoon at a time in water—no more than one tablespoon an hour (3 teaspoons make up a tablespoon). This acts as a preventive during an epidemic. If you are caught in a flu epidemic you will also want to read the recipe listed in the *Cayenne Pepper* section and the cinnamon bark preventive.

Vinegar of the Four Thieves

2   quarts apple cider vinegar
2   tablespoons lavender
2   tablespoons rosemary
2   tablespoons sage
2   tablespoons wormwood
2   tablespoons rue
2   tablespoons mint
2   tablespoons garlic buds

Combine the dried herbs (except the garlic), and steep in the vinegar in the sun for two weeks. Strain and rebottle.

Label. Add several cloves of garlic. Close lid. When garlic has steeped for several days, strain out. Melt paraffin wax around the lid to preserve the contents, or add 4 ounces of glycerine for preservation.

Note dosage above.

Modern Antiepidemic Vinegar ★

1 quart apple cider vinegar
1 pound garlic buds for 8 ounces expressed juice
8 ounces comfrey root
4 ounces oak bark
4 ounces marshmallow root
4 ounces mullein flowers
4 ounces rosemary flowers
4 ounces lavender flowers
4 ounces wormwood
4 ounces black walnut leaves
About 12 ounces glycerine

Make separate teas of each of the herbs. First soak each ounce of herb in clean spring water. After about half a day, simmer each herb separately for ten minutes. Steep for a half hour. Strain out, simmer again, and reduce each herb so that it is concentrated. Press garlic buds into 8 ounces of concentrated juice. Add 12 ounces of glycerine to preserve it. Place in a *large* bottle. *Label.* Close. You may want to add paraffin for additional preservation power.

Dosage: 1–3 teaspoons during epidemics, or 1 teaspoon per hour if someone in the family is ill with a communicable disease. Dilute with water if too strong to take, or use added to hot herbal tea.

Herb Vinegars for Facial, Bath, or Salad

(1)

1 quart apple cider vinegar
4 tablespoons dried herbs (or 2 tablespoons fresh herbs)

Place vinegar in a ceramic or glass pot. Bring to a brief boil. Turn off heat. Add herbs. Pour into vinegar jar. Use leftover vinegar for body wash or addition to bath.

(2)

1   quart apple cider vinegar
1   handful fresh mint or tarragon (or 3 tablespoons dried mint)

Wash mint, bruise leaves well, and pack into jar. Cover tightly, and let stand two weeks. Strain out the herbs. (If dried mint is used, first simmer the vinegar, bring to a boil, and then pour over the mint.)

(3)

½   pint apple cider vinegar
1   ounce rose petals
½   pint rosewater

Mix and steep for two weeks. If preferred, white vinegar can be substituted for apple cider vinegar.

(4)

½   pint vinegar (apple cider or white)
1   ounce several different kinds of aromatic flowers (examples: lavender, sweet violet, rosemary)

Mix and steep for two weeks.

OINTMENT

An ointment is a soothing, healing, slightly oily or fatty substance into which the essence of a healing plant has been dissolved. Basically this is accomplished by heating the fat or oil with the plant until it loses its normal color and the oil or fat has absorbed the healing chemical principles. The plant is then strained out, and beeswax is added to harden the ointment. Preservatives such as drops of tincture of benzoin, poplar bud tincture, or glycerine are optional additions. If you make ointments in small batches and keep them tightly lidded and closed with paraffin wax, they don't decompose.

The Base

Pork Lard   This is a traditional folk, herbal, and pharmaceutical base for ointments. Purify it by simmering and straining. It has healing abilities even without the addition of herbs, but, then, so do a lot of fats and oils. It is said to have great drawing power, but despite this undoubted virtue, its accessibility, and inexpensive price, I prefer the following fats and oils.

Lanolin   I use a purified, liquefied anhydrous lanolin. Lanolin, the substance washed from the wool of sheep, comes in many levels of purity, so the results vary depending on the product. This oil is the closest to skin oil. Some people are allergic to lanolin, however. If you think you may be allergic, purchase small amounts and only the purest of the products.

Neutral Oil Bases—Almond Oil, Cocoa Butter, Wheat Germ, Vitamin E   Almond oil is a more neutral base than lanolin, as is wheat germ oil, cocoa butter, or vitamin E. If you have no other product available, or if you are applying mashed garlic to the soles of the feet in the antiflu procedure, Vaseline may be used, but is listed here for emergency purposes only.

Thickeners

All ointments must contain one substance that will thicken the final product. Lanolin is a thickener, as is cocoa butter. Both are nonsticky and mix well with most other oils.

Cocoa butter is available in 2-ounce lipstick-shaped containers and can be purchased in drugstores. In addition to its thickening abilities, cocoa butter is useful for its healing potential, for internal suppositories (it melts at body temperature), skin lotions (lovely during the summer to increase light tanning), and for ointments.

Purified lanolin is available through Caswell-Massey, Kiehl's, and possibly through local botanical sources.

Other useful but sticky thickeners are glycerine, honey, or liquid lecithin. In addition, various powdered resins and gum swell up and thicken when first soaked in cold water, then simmered in gentle boiling water, and added to preparations. Agar-agar and Irish moss are seaweed thickeners. Green apples provide an excellent acid fruit pectin that is a good addition to skin creams and ointments.

Hardeners

While any of the above sticky and nonsticky thickeners will help swell a product and keep it emulsified (so that it doesn't separate into parts), you will still need some wax to harden a cold cream or ointment. Beeswax is perfect. However, it is terribly expensive on the open market. I therefore combine beeswax with paraffin wax.

Make-Ahead Wax Portions

It is fun to make ointments on the spur of the moment or when you have picked a plant you want to work with. Since it is difficult to break off just the right size chunk of beeswax for small batches of ointment, I devised this make-ahead table-spoon-portion mold.

Collect two egg cartons. Take off the tops. With aluminum foil, work out a layer across the indented top, and gently depress the thin foil into a mold that will easily take a tablespoon of the melted wax.

Heat a small chunk of wax in a nonaluminum pot. With a cold, clean silver or stainless steel soup spoon, lift out a full measure of the melted wax. Place it piping hot in the aluminum mold. Wipe the spoon with a paper towel. Rinse in cold water, and dry the spoon. Repeat the process until you have twenty-four (or more) tablespoon portions. When the wax hardens, lift out, and place in box or plastic bag. It will keep indefinitely and is easily cut in half if necessary.

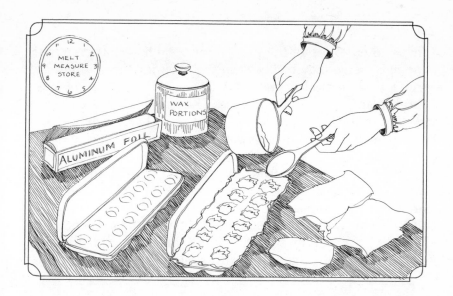

To Make a Simple Ointment

8   ounces lard by weight
2   ounces or 4 tablespoons wax

Melt wax, add lard gradually, and stir until cool. This is the basis for most old-fashioned pharmaceutical ointments. It can be varied by using a cooking oil, such as safflower or olive, or sweet almond oil or avocado.

Herbal Ointments

The following herbs made up excellent healing ointments: goldenseal, goldenseal and slippery elm, plantain, pot marigold *(Calendula officinalis)*, juniper berries, comfrey root, leaf, cucumber, yarrow leaves, plantain leaves, marigold flowers, arnica flowers, meadowsweet, chickweed, lady's mantle, wintergreen, eucalyptus, elderflower.

Basic Recipe

Crush fresh or dried herbs and simmer with lard, lanolin, wheat germ oil, vitamin E oil, safflower, almond oil, and so on. Simmer on top of the stove for several hours. If preferred, the ingredients may be baked in the oven for several hours. (I prefer this method.) Strain out the sizzling (and sometimes burnt) plant material. Place in jar. The ointment is ready when the lard or the lanolin hardens. If it doesn't harden, reheat and add a small amount of beeswax depending on the size of the preparation.

To make a very strong preparation, strain off the first batch of herbs and add another handful or batch to the strained liquid. Boil again to a watery decoction, and add olive oil until the water has evaporated. Strain off the plant. Add beeswax or resin to solidify. These must be added in hot melted condition so that they mix uniformly in the ointment.

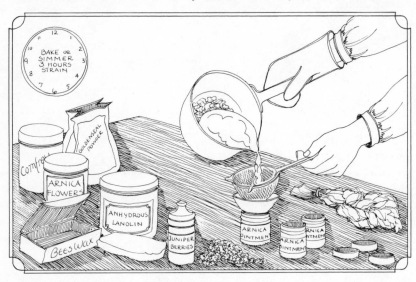

Plantain Liquefied Ointment

> 2½ cups fresh plantain leaves
> 1½ cups wheat germ oil
> ½   cup honey

Mix the wheat germ oil and the honey in a blender, making sure the blades are covered with the oil. Add fresh plantain leaves. Scrape out the preparation with a spatula. Place in a labeled bottle or jar.

To solidify, add 2½ tablespoons or more of hot, melted beeswax.

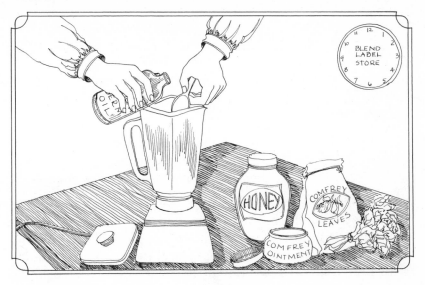

Sore Leg Ointment

> 1   handful chickweed
> 1   handful red rose leaves
> 1   pint oil (any)

Cook the chickweed and the red rose leaves together in the oil on top of the stove or in the oven. After one to three hours, strain out the herbs. Use as liquid ointment on sore legs.

Juniper Berry Ointment   This ointment is useful for wounds, itching, scratches, scars from burns, hangnails, and festering sores.

Collect the berries from the garden or the wild just as they are getting ripe.

> 2   cups juniper berries
> 2   cups oil (olive, peanut, wheat germ, lanolin)
> 2–3 tablespoons   (or   more   if   necessary) beeswax

Soak the berries overnight. Strain out the water. Simmer the berries in the oil and take care that they do not burn. Heat the wax in a separate container. Strain out the berries. Add the melted wax while the preparation is hot. Since each batch has a slightly different consistency, the amount of wax must be added by eye after the hardening process has started. If necessary, reheat and add additional melted wax.

Golden Wound Paste

Equal amounts slippery elm bark powder and goldenseal root powder
1   tablespoon olive oil (or spring water)

Just mix the two powders together to make a paste. Add the olive oil or the spring water, and apply on a cloth to a wound. Attach to the body with a bandage or elastic binding. Later wash the wound with sage tea. If the wound is festering with pus, roll and press down the ridges of a white cabbage leaf, and/or attach or mash some banana, and apply to suppurating area.

The combination of the slippery elm (soothing), goldenseal (antiseptic and healing), sage (cleansing), and cabbage and/or banana is very effective.

Cucumber Ointment

1   pound (7 pounds for a large quantity) cucumber
3¼ ounces (24 ounces for large quantity) pure lard
2¼ ounces (15 ounces for large quantity) veal suet

Grate the washed cucumbers into a pulp, or use blender or food processor. Strain the juice. Cut suet into small pieces, heat over a water bath until the fat is melted out from the membrane, and then add the lard. When melted, strain through the muslin into an earthen vessel capable of holding up to 1 gallon (if the larger quantity is utilized). Stir until thickening starts. Add ⅓ of the juice.

Beat with a spatula until the odor has been wholly extracted. Put into jar and cover. Heat in a water bath until the fatty matter separates from the juice. Strain off the green coagulum floating on the surface. Put jar in a cool place to solidify.

The crude ointment is then separated from the watery liquid on which it floats, melted and strained, and placed in glass jars which must be kept sealed. Add a layer of rosewater on the surface to help preserve it. Rosewater may also be added to make this preparation creamy and white. This is a most healing and cleansing cream.

The very best, and oldest, of professional cucumber creams is made by the Caswell-Massey firm which maintains a worldwide mail-order business. Culpeper in London also has an excellent cream.

Emergency Ointment Combine wheat germ oil and honey. Apply to sore, bruise, or wound. If you have tinctures of comfrey, calendula, St. John's wort, or mullein, add 5–15 drops of the tincture to oil and honey.

Ointment for Painful Sores

> 8 ounces vegetable glycerine
> 2 ounces white oak bark powder

Heat together in top of double boiler for thirty minutes. Cool, strain, bottle, and label.

Soothing Soaps Napier's in Edinburgh produces a famous healing slippery elm soap. Culpeper in London, Caswell-Massey in New York and elsewhere, all produce other skin-healing soaps.

SUPPOSITORIES

In the main, suppositories are solid cylindrical objects designed to help evacuate the bowels by slightly irritating the mucous membranes of the rectum. Shaped solid glycerine or soap cylinders will accomplish this. This will stimulate bowel movements and can replace irrigation by water (enema).

In folk medicine there is an ancient tradition of insertion of healing and/or astringent herbs to topically relieve specific rectal or vaginal pain or discharges. One such herb that comes to mind is the powdered bark of the slippery elm which has been used for centuries to help overcome many vaginal problems. Here, a small amount of tepid water is added to make a rather thick paste which is then molded into 1-inch cylinders. Several are inserted into the vagina, and leakage is prevented by use of a sanitary napkin. After three days the vagina is douched with water to cleanse it.

In the late 1880's, Sir J. Y. Simpson of Edinburgh discovered that cocoa butter had unique attributes for medicated suppositories (pessaries). These suppositories are available by prescription at the advice of your physician. The following is my grandmother's version of such a remedy, and while it should not replace prescriptions advised by your physician, the recipes may prove to be useful in remote areas, or during emergencies when professional attention is not available.

Cocoa Butter

Cocoa butter is made from the expressed oil of the chocolate nut (ground seeds of Theobroma Cacao). It is usually used for cosmetics, and soothes skin affected by either windburn or sunburn. It can be purchased in one-ounce round cylinders in drug stores. It has a tallow consistency, a white to yellow color, is bland, healing, and has a most agreeable smell. It is ideal for medicated insertion into both the vagina and/or rectum (except in the case of an allergy to topical use of cocoa butter) because it melts quickly when heated, combines readily with powdered, grated herbs, and is quickly shaped into pencil-shaped suppository cylinders. Once inserted into the rectum or vagina, the combined cocoa butter and herb has the advantage of melting slowly at body temperature. Depending on the internal need, either healing or astringent herbs may be added. Astringent herbs help to clear up discharges. Use pads of absorbent cotton or a sanitary napkin to catch discharges.

Preparation

Grate, or grind with a mortar and pestle, either such healing herbs as comfrey root or leaf, or marshmallow root, or such astringent herbs as witch hazel, or yellow dock or bayberry. Drops of the tincture or extracts of these herbs may also be used. My grandmother used about ten drops of the tincture or extract, or a teaspoon of the herb for every tablespoon of the cocoa butter (two tablespoons for every ounce). These are melted together in the top of a double boiler.

Making a Mold   Before melting the powdered herb and cocoa butter cylinders, prepare a disposable aluminum foil mold. Indent a heavy duty aluminum wrap into 2 to 2½ inch long and ¾ of an inch wide sections. Immediately before the melting process place this improvised mold in the refrigerator. Melt the cocoa butter and the previously selected herb or herbs. Take the mold out of the refrigerator and either dust it with lycopodium powder or brush it with a light coating of olive oil. Pour the melted substance into the mold. The cold will immediately chill the melted material; the powder or olive oil will prevent sticking.

Shape the material, as soon as possible after it hardens, into pencil shapes; wider at the bottom for rectal insertion; or a ¾ inch base and tapering shape for vaginal insertion. Store the medicinal suppositories, or pessaries, in an opaque, labeled container.

Suppository

> 3   ounces cocoa butter
> 1   ounce powdered herb (witch hazel, bayberry, or yellow dock)

Simmer the herb and cocoa butter in the top of a double boiler. Stir and watch until the preparation seems pliable and

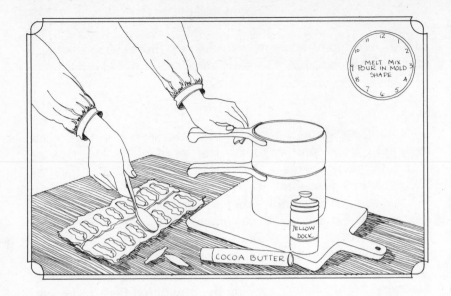

almost firm. Pour out into foil mold. Roll into 2 to 2½-inch cylinder shape with center tapering slightly outward.

Hemorrhoids

Insert suppository in rectum after each bowel movement.

White Vaginal Discharge

Insert suppository every other day. Use sanitary napkin to catch any leakage. On between days, douche with diluted apple cider vinegar, diluted acidophilus and water, or diluted yellow dock tea. Note other comments on vaginal discharges in the book.

Internal Cleansing Program

Insert suppository in vagina for two days at a time. Use sanitary napkin to catch excess leakage. Every third day, douche with lukewarm yellow dock tea. Continue program for about a week. Acid wastes will be flushed out through vagina and rectum.

LIP BALM

Preparation of Oil

2–4 tablespoons rose petals (or marigold
    petals)
1   cup almond oil

Use sun to extract the fragrance of the petals into the oil.
Fill the jar loosely with the petals, and slowly drizzle oil over
them. Fill to within 1 inch of the top of the jar. Close jar and
label. Place in the sun for five days in summer, or three days in
a very hot climate, or fifteen days in the winter sun. Strain
during the warm part of the day. Using fine mesh, press the
herb petals to extract all the oil.

Preparation of Balm

    As above, warm rose oil
1   tablespoon beeswax
1   teaspoon honey
1   teaspoon vanilla extract
1   teaspoon vitamin E oil
1   teaspoon aloe vera gel

Warm the oil in an improvised double-boiler arrangement.
Stir continuously. Add 1 tablespoon of beeswax. Add the
honey, vanilla extract, vitamin E oil, and aloe vera gel. Stir hot
into wide-mouthed ointment container. Close with tight lid.
The balm will soon harden. This is very nourishing for the lips.

Lip Balm #2

Another healing lip balm is prepared by combining 7
ounces of cocoa butter, 1 ounce of yellow wax, a teaspoon each
of balsam of Peru and benzoic acid; straining; adding a little

rose oil, and, when nearly cool, a quarter of a teaspoon of glycerine.

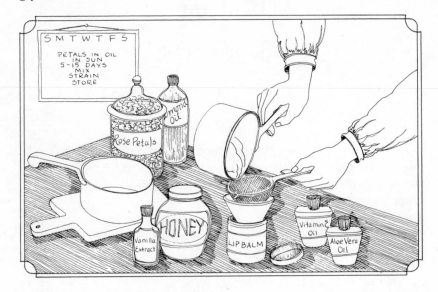

ESSENCE

There are several ways to make home essences and to extract oil from aromatic or high-oil-yield flowers:

1. Obtain a minute amount of an oil by the evaporation of flower petals in a tightly stoppered glass container, which stands for several days in the sun.

2. Use that oil or commercially prepared aromatic or bland vegetable oil as a base to capture the aroma of other highly scented herbs.

3. Combine finely crushed herb powders with, or without, the addition of commercially prepared herbal oils, and dissolve these powders (and possibly the oils) into a strong alcohol medium. The entire preparation is then passed through a conical parchment filter. This is sometimes called a "spirit." Commercial peppermint, lavender compound, and lemon essence are prepared in this way.

Some Highly Scented Herbs for Oil Preparation

Camelia	Peppermint
Cardamom	Red saunders
Chamomile	Rosemary
Geranium	Sweet cicely
Jasmine	Tonquin beans
Lavender	Vanilla
Lemon	Vetiver

A Home Flower Essence

A pint of aromatic flower petals will yield about a tablespoon of aromatic oil. Pick fresh flowers early in the morning before the sun comes up. Take off the stems, and press about a hundred or more into a small, sterilized jar. Whatever the size of the jar, pack the petals tightly. Close the lid. Place the jar in the sun.

No water is needed. The sun evaporates the oils and water from the flowers and, as they shrivel, the oil falls to the bottom of the jar. In a day or so you will notice the drops of moisture and oil. Watch the jar, for as soon as the moisture stops dripping, you must retrieve the precious liquid. While it isn't a matter of moments, it is interesting to see that nature will then reverse the process and allow the flowers to reabsorb the lost oils and water. Take out the top layer of flowers with a tweezer or chopsticks, and press the bottom petals to squeeze out the lower level of oil.

You will need a funnel to catch every drop. Enclose in a dark, tightly stoppered glass jar that has been sterilized to eliminate any previous odor. Preserve by adding a few drops of tincture of benzoin, a perfect preservative for oil, ointment, tincture, sachet, and potpourri.

Rose Oil

If you grow roses you can make small amounts of your own rare, expensive, true rose oil. Use equal parts of rose oil and glycerine to make an elegant, rich hand and face lotion. Use less glycerine if you don't like it thick. Glycerine is another excellent preservative for oils, ointments, tinctures, and other herbal preparations. There is now a vegetable glycerine on the market.

Skin-Absorbing Oils

Use any of the following oils to make up an aromatic skin oil that will be absorbed quickly:

Corn, safflower, sesame, sunflower, walnut, and wheat germ.

Nonabsorbent Massage Oils

These saturated fats are all softening agents that will not be easily absorbed by the skin: sweet almond, avocado, coconut, cocoa butter, olive, apricot kernel, peanut, and palm.

Making Herb Oil

Decide on the oil base and the flower petal(s) you wish to use. (You may use one or more varieties.) One successful, easy combination consists of lavender flowers, rose petals, chamomile flowers, elder flowers, and orris root powder (fixative).

> 2–3 cups almond oil (or any oil on list)
> 1   tablespoon dried lavender flowers
> 1   tablespoon fresh or dried rose petals
> 1   tablespoon fresh or dried chamomile flowers
> 1   tablespoon dried elder flowers
> 1   tablespoon orris root powder (fixative)

Fill jar loosely with the herbs. Sprinkle the orris root powder in the jar. Slowly pour the oil over the herbs. Make sure all the air bubbles are out. Fill the oil to within an inch of the top of the jar. Close the jar. In summer, put this jar in the sun for about five days (some hot areas may need even less time). In the winter, place the jar in the sun for fifteen days. Shake each day.

At the end of the alloted time, during the very hot part of the day, slowly drizzle the oil through a fine mesh strainer into a funnel at the mouth of a small, sterilized jar. Press the herbs as you go along. Repeat the straining process until the oil is free of herbs.

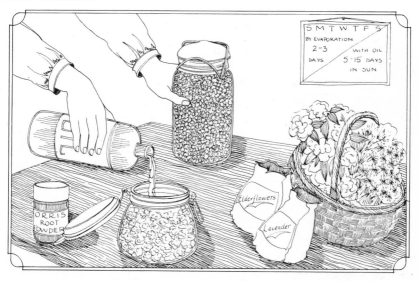

Massage Oil

Herbs to Soften and Heal Skin Comfrey, calendula (pot marigold), slippery elm, St. John's wort, marshmallow, flaxseed, fenugreek, psyllium seed, aloe vera. Follow herb oil directions or rosemary massage oil directions.

Herbs to Aid Sore Muscles Arnica, lavender, rosemary, St. John's wort, calendula, chamomile, comfrey, mullein flowers, wintergreen, eucalyptus, camphor, ginger (the last four will heat the area), juniper berries. Follow herb oil directions or rosemary massage oil directions.

Rosemary Massage Oil

2   cups peanut oil (or any oil on massage list)
1   tablespoon hydrous lanolin
1   tablespoon vitamin E oil
1   tablespoon dried lavender flowers
1   tablespoon dried rose petals
1   tablespoon dried chamomile flowers
3   tablespoons dried rosemary flowers
¼   teaspoon tincture of benzoin (fixative)

Follow the directions for herb oil.

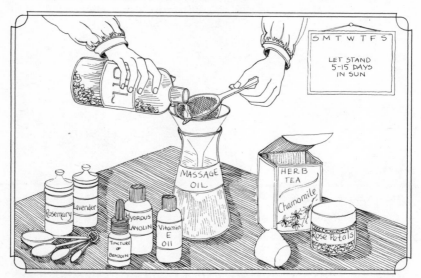

Juniper Berry Massage Oil [for ointment]   This is a healing lotion which is also useful for itching problems, wounds, scratches, and back problems.

Use dried juniper berries or fresh ripening berries. Use larger amounts of the berries for extra healing power.

2   cups juniper berries
2   cups peanut oil
     Several drops per teaspoon aromatic oil (optional), depending on personal taste

This oil has a marvelous healing effect.

Soak the berries in a small amount of water overnight. This will get them mushy. Put the water aside, and simmer the berries and oil together. Watch closely to avoid burning. Strain out the berries. Use the oil. Note: Adding heated beeswax or paraffin to this oil will make it into a healing ointment.

Spirit of Lavender

1 part essential oil of lavender
49 parts brandy

You can use 1 drop of the oil to 49 drops of brandy or, by eye, drop of oil to ¾ a teaspoon of brandy. (A drop is a *minim*, or a sixtieth part of a fluid dram. One fluid dram equals 1 teaspoon.)

Use this preparation in ½ to 1 teaspoon doses set in a tablespoon of water or milk. This preparation is useful for palpitation, nervousness, faintness, giddiness, spasms, colic, flatulence, and, moreover, somewhat rallies a flagging spirit.

To Preserve Flowers That Are to be Used for Aromatic Waters or Potpourri

Fresh flowers are preferred, but if you pick a huge batch of aromatic flowers and know you cannot get to them immediately, you can preserve them intact for up to two years by first packing them firmly in wide-mouthed bottles. Do not crush them. Pour glycerine over the flowers until they are covered. Close the jar. Elder, rose, and orange flowers, for instance, can be preserved in this way. Flowers can also be packed in one third their weight of common salt to preserve them. This is useful for a potpourri blend of several aromatic herbs.

EXTRACT

Extracts are solid substances resulting from the evaporation of the solution of vegetable principles. The extract is obtained in three ways: (1) by expressing the juice of fresh plants (as in *Succus calendula*, the juice of the pot marigold), (2) by using a solvent such as alcohol, or (3) by simmering a plant tea and reducing it to a thickened state. The latter is accomplished by simmering a plant (an example could be cloves) and by repeating the process until most of the water used has evaporated. This is a decoction. This gives you a distillation of the most active principles in the plant. Add ¼ teaspoon of alcohol (brandy, gin, or vodka will do), glycerine, or tincture of benzoin to preserve the extract.

Many plants are commercially available in extract form. The Father Kneipp brand of plant juices is available from many gourmet shops.

The expressed juices of borage, chamomile, celery, dandelion, hawthorn, horsetail, melissa, nettle, paprika, parsley, pumpkin, rosemary, thyme, valerian, watercress, wormwood, yarrow, and beets are available from Bio-Nutritional Products, P.O. Box 389, Harrison, N.Y. 10528.

Extract Distillation of Cloves

1 tablespoon cloves
1½ cups water

Boil until it is a syrup. Repeat three times.

This is useful in tiny doses and, on rare occasions, for sleep problems. Use a teaspoon of the distillation in a cup of hot herbal chamomile or linden tea. The stronger the distillation, the more sedative and sleep-producing it becomes.

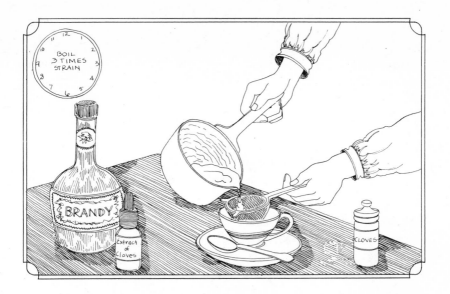

SYRUP

Medicinal syrups are formed when sugar is incorporated with vegetable infusions, decoctions, expressed juices, fermented liquors, or simple water solutions. Sometimes tinctures are added to a simple syrup, and the alcohol is evaporated. The tincture is occasionally combined with sugar and gently heated, or exposed to the sun until the alcohol is evaporated, and the syrup then prepared with the impregnated sugar and water. Refined sugar makes a clearer and better-flavored syrup. Any simple syrup can be preserved by substituting glycerine for a certain portion of the syrup. Always make syrups in small quantities.

Some Syrups and Jellies

Simple Syrup

35 ounces refined sugar
20 fluid ounces distilled water

Dissolve the sugar in the water over heat. Raise the temperature to the boiling point, and strain the solution while hot. Then add enough extra distilled water through the strainer to make the syrup measure 2 pints and 12 fluid ounces.

Mulberry Syrup

1   pint mulberry juice
2   pounds refined sugar
2½ fluid ounces rectified spirit (vodka or gin)

Heat the mulberry juice to the boiling point and, when it has cooled, filter it. Dissolve the filtered sugar in the filtered liquid with gentle heat, and add the vodka, gin, or rectified spirit. Let the strained juice stand from eight to fifteen hours, and let it ferment. The juice separates into two portions. The upper third is clear. Separate this section by straining, and make into syrup by adding water.

Rose Hip Jelly

1   pint rose hips
     Enough water to make rose hips float
1   pint sugar to each pint rose hips

Take a large quantity of well-ripened rose hips. Wash them in a colander, and set them out to dry. Slit them lengthwise, and remove the hairs and pips with a sharp penknife (you can save the pips for fruit butter). Weigh the hips and put them in a pan filled with enough water to float them. Add a pint of sugar for each pint of fruit. Boil the mixture together until it is quite soft. Strain off the liquid, and boil it again for a few minutes. Pour it into jars and seal. Label.

Second Method: Start as above, but instead of soaking the rose hips, cook them in very little water. Then strain off the juice. Measure it. Boil it up again for ten minutes and add 1 pint of warmed sugar for each pint of juice. Cook until jelly sets. Jar it and seal.

To Make a Jelly into a Medicated Syrup: Add 2½ pints of vodka or rectified spirit for every pint of the juice.

A Syrup with Fluid Extract

> 10–15 drops bayberry root fluid extract
> 1   spoonful honey

Mix and swallow slowly to aid sore throat.

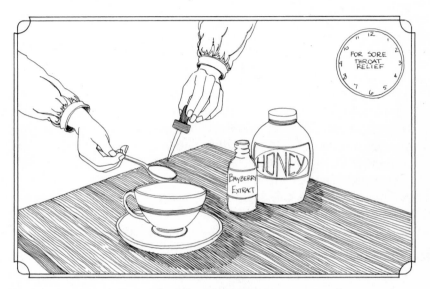

ELECTUARY

When powders are mixed with syrup, honey, brown sugar, or glycerine to produce a more pleasant taste or to render them more convenient for internal use, they are called electuaries. These are rarely prepared in advance, but are done on the spur of the moment as needed. Different substances require different proportions of syrup. Light vegetable powders usually require twice their weight, gum resins two thirds their weight, mineral substances about half their weight.

If an electuary is made up in advance and it hardens, add more syrup. If it swells up and emits gas, merely beat it up again in the mortar.

To Use Tea as a Syrup

Prepare any herbal tea, and simmer it down for a longer time so that very little of the water is left. Add 1 ounce of glycerin. Seal the syrup in a jar, as if it were fruit, by using a paraffin wax enclosure.

MARSHMALLOW SWEETS

My grandmother knew the marvelous Romanian gypsy technique of chewing marshmallow leaves and uniting with saliva for a truly healing poultice. She also made marshmallow sweets with sugar, root, gum, and a touch of egg white. While she usually made it up into big batches, here is my small-batch reconstruction of the recipe. Of particular importance is the quality of the roots—make sure they aren't moldy or too woody. Marshmallow gives off almost twice its own weight of mucilaginous gel when placed in water.

      4 tablespoons marshmallow roots
     28 tablespoons refined sugar
     20 tablespoons gum tragacanth (or gum ara-
          bic)
          Water of orange flowers (for aroma or
          instead of plain water)
      2 cups water
    1–2 egg whites, well beaten

Make up a tea of marshmallow roots by simmering in a pint of water for twenty to thirty minutes. Add additional water if it simmers down. Strain out the roots. Heat the gum and marshmallow decoction (water) in a double boiler until they are dissolved together. Strain with pressure. Stir in the sugar as quickly as possible. When dissolved, add the well-beaten egg white(s), stirring constantly, but take off the fire and continue to stir. Lay out on a flat surface. Let cool, and cut into smaller pieces.

CONSERVES

When you add sugar and beat it into a plant substance, the result is called a conserve. The sugar helps the plant to resist decomposition. But the action of bruising and cutting the plant may also take away its medicinal value. Use refined sugar in fine powder.

This process, or jam-making, is useful in preserving berries of medicinal value. (Also see *Marigold Conserve.*)

SPROUT CANDY

There is no sugar in this recipe.

> 2 cups each dried figs, dates, prunes, apricots
> 1 cup wheat berry sprouts
> Water

Chop the fruit into small pieces. Put the fruit and sprouts through a food grinder. Add enough water to make a thick paste. Roll the paste into balls. The balls can be rolled into coconut, carob powder, wheat germ, sesame seeds, etc. Wrap in waxed paper, and refrigerate or freeze.

LOZENGES

Lozenges or troches are small, dry, solid plant powders combined with sugar and mucilage (marshmallow root, slippery elm bark, comfrey root, or gum mucilage such as gum tragacanth—the best mucilage).

Spread herb powder with sugar and form a paste. Spread marble slab with sugar, and roll paste into a flat cake. Cover top layer with sugar and cornstarch. Divide into small cakes with a knife. Place the cakes on white paper, and expose to the air for twelve hours. Next, place in dry, airy area. When the small lozenges are perfectly dry, place on a sieve to separate the sugar and starch. Enclose them in bottles.

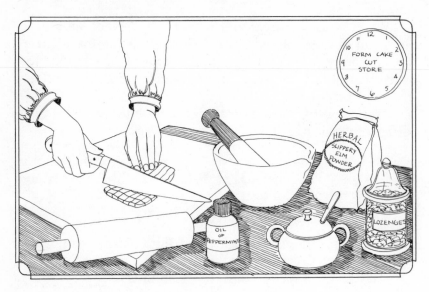

Oil of Peppermint Lozenges

12 drops oil of peppermint
2 ounces refined sugar
Enough mucilage of tragacanth to help make it into a paste

Rub the oil of peppermint with the sugar until they are thoroughly mixed; then form a mass with the mucilage of tragacanth. Roll flat. Cut into lozenges or troches.

To Make Mucilage of Tragacanth

1 ounce tragacanth
1 pint boiling water

Soak the tragacanth and stir for twenty-four hours. Beat the mixture into uniform consistency, and force through a muslin strainer. The mixture must be beaten, as only part of tragacanth is soluble in water and, thus, doesn't form a uniform solution.

When kept too long, it can decompose.

PILLS

Powdered herbs may be enclosed in gelatine capsules and swallowed with water. This is also useful when combining several herbs or when the taste or smell is too strong to drink in tea form.

To preserve pills, roll in powdered licorice root or lycopodium powder, and place in a perforated tin box. The lycopodium does not attract moisture. Add additional licorice powder if the pills are too soft.

I sometimes roll pieces of cut herb in cream cheese to make a quick herbal pill.

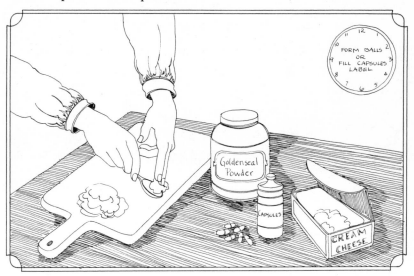

INSECT REPELLENTS

There are a great many common garden herbs and culinary herbs that can be used safely for indoor and outdoor help in repelling insects. Among the everyday culinary herbs are sage, cayenne, rosemary, and basil. Cinnamon, nutmeg, mace, and caraway seeds can be made into a potpourri or pomander ball. Tansy will repel ants. Dried root of khus khus is an insect repellent that can be used in clothes drawers; sage leaves will deter moths, cockroaches, and rodents. Chamomile flowers can be made into a tea and pressed on the body for an effective antimosquito aid; cayenne pepper is disliked by insects; and various herbs and herb oils may be safely combined to make other potent repellents.

Insect Repellent Oil   This preparation is terrific and has even been used by friends in South and Central American jungles; however, some people may be allergic to these oils, so use with caution.

> 1   ounce rue oil
> 1   ounce rosemary oil
> 1   ounce basil oil   .
> 1   ounce wormwood oil

Combine in small bottles to carry in your pocket. Label.

Insecticide

> ½   teaspoon rosemary oil
> ½   pint light beer

Combine and use as spray or lotion.

Another good repellent:

> 2   tablespoons rosemary powder
> 2   tablespoons wormwood leaf powder

Combine and place in areas of the room, closets, or drawers to repel insects.

Sage leaves will deter moths, cockroaches, and rodents.

Outdoor Sage-Rosemary Candle   Crumble sage and rosemary leaves. Add dry grass and crumbled white wax. Put a match to the ingredients for an outdoor repellent. This smoke will keep away mosquitoes.

Note: chamomile, wormwood, rue, lavender oil, and pennyroyal—all are useful in this type of outdoor candle.

Fumigator Place a tablespoon of red pepper on a bottle lid. Place over a Sterno, or candle-type food warmer, and light the underneath candle to heat the lid. Allow the pepper to fume. Close the room. Repeat as often as necessary.

Head Lice

1   pint white wine (or white vinegar)
3   tablespoons rue

Crumble rue into the white wine (or white vinegar). Steep as long as possible—two weeks is best but, if in a hurry, use before. This is potent for body lice, skin parasites, or as a ringworm lotion.

Sage Bunches Many insects dislike sage. Tie garden or wild sage in bunches, and hang around the house, around outdoor porches and terraces, or hang from trees in frequently used outdoor spots.

Moth Preventive

2   tablespoons cloves
2   tablespoons caraway seeds
2   tablespoons nutmeg
2   tablespoons mace
2   tablespoons cinnamon
2   tablespoons tonquin beans
12   tablespoons orris root powder (fixative)

Grind all the herbs together. Add and mix in orris root powder. Place in cheesecloth or cotton bags in closets, drawers, and trunks.

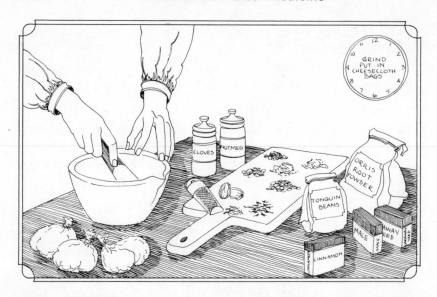

Rodent Repellent Rats hate peppermint. Old-time rat catchers closed all but one exit in a house, cellar, or barn, placed peppermint oil on cloths, and the rats rushed out and were caught in the bag held over the exit.

On the opposite side of the coin, rats love valerian root.

HERB DEODORANT

½ teaspoon cloves
1 teaspoon myrrh
1 tablespoon coriander seeds
1 teaspoon cassia
2 tablespoons lavender flowers
1 teaspoon thyme

Grind up all the ingredients in a small hand mill or with a mortar and pestle. I use this and similar blends as a bath powder, or under the arms as a deodorant. Because there is always a possibility of skin sensitivity with topical use of dried herbs, test your skin reaction by using only tiny amounts at a time. Experiment with other aromatic combinations, too.

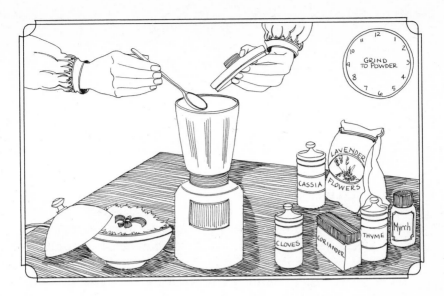

DOUCHE

Douches are useful in overcoming specific internal problems but should not be used on a regular basis as they may reduce natural protection. For persistent problems see your health professional or gynecologist.

Ovarian Infection

1. Prepare a rosemary tea with 1 tablespoon dried rosemary to 2 quarts boiling water. Steep. Cool. Use for seven days as a vaginal douche.

2. Red Raspberry douche: Use as directed above.

Discharges

Use apple cider vinegar douches for trichomonas infection.

Use powder from acidophilus capsule plus water for douche when there is a yeast infection.

Yeast Infection Douche

1   teaspoon chamomile
1   teaspoon powdered goldenseal
1   teaspoon-1 cup comfrey root or leaf
2   tablespoons apple cider vinegar
1   tablet acidophilus, liquefied
2   tablespoons witch hazel liquid
2   quarts water

Add 1 cup boiling water to chamomile flowers and goldenseal powder. Steep fifteen minutes. Strain out the flowers. Add 1 cup of strained comfrey leaf or comfrey root tea. Steep. Mix apple cider vinegar, liquefied acidophilus ingredients, witch hazel. Make up 2 quarts. Douche.

Use every other day for a week. This is very effective and should help control the infection.

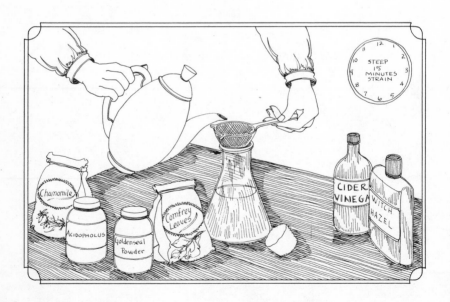

BREATH SWEETENERS, MOUTHWASH, THROAT GARGLES

Herbal Breath Sweeteners

Many Indian restaurants serve large fat fennel seeds as an after-dinner breath sweetener. This use of seeds after eating is also a custom in many Near and Far Eastern countries. Mace seeds are sucked in some countries, as are star anise seeds. Angelica seeds are sucked, and in some places nutmeg is both chewed and sucked (not advisable). Whole cloves, calamus root pieces, peppermint leaves and oil, and cinnamon and caraway seeds are other herbal breath sweeteners.

To Make a Mouthwash

Use pint bottles of sherry or small amounts of leftover white wine, and adjust the herbal ingredients according to the amount of wine on hand. Leftover wine doesn't always last too long—it actually depends on the type of wine and the grape, so don't make up big batches unless you intend to keep the mouthwash in the refrigerator. My mouthwashes with sherry have always lasted a long time.

Mint Mouthwash

½ teaspoon peppermint, dried
½ teaspoon thyme leaves, dried
½ teaspoon cloves, crushed
½ teaspoon nutmeg, fresh-grated
½ pint sherry
10 drops oil of peppermint

Use any inexpensive sherry, and adjust herbs accordingly. Steep herbs only for a week to ten days. Strain out the herbs. Add the peppermint oil drops. Label.

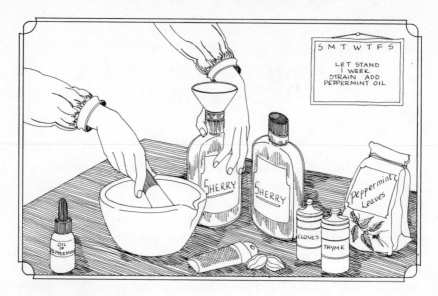

Myrrh Mouthwash

3   drops tincture of myrrh
1   glass water

Add several drops of tincture of myrrh to water for a cleansing but bitter-tasting mouthwash. Myrrh is very antiseptic and will immediately ease pain of mouth sores. A very small amount of about equal portions of goldenseal root powder and tincture of myrrh in water makes an excellent mouthwash for canker sores and often controls them overnight.

Spicy Wine or Mouthwash

1   bottle wine, white or red
2   ounces (several small bruised sticks) cinnamon
6   peppercorns
½   nutmeg, bruised or grated
2   tablespoons or a half handful rosemary

Place all the herbs and peppercorns in the wine. Steep for two weeks. Strain. Label. Keep corked.

Leftover wine may be used; just adjust the herbs accordingly.

Gargle and Mouthwash

> 2 cups apple cider vinegar
> 1 cup water
> 1 handful wintergreen leaves

Soak the wintergreen leaves, or leaves and flowers, in the apple cider vinegar for twenty-four hours. Add the water to dilute. Strain out the wintergreen. Close lid. Label.

Use warm for gargle. Use cold for mouthwash.

Sage-Cayenne Gargle

> ½ pint sage tea
> 2 teaspoons honey
> 2 tablespoons salt
> 2 tablespoons vinegar (apple)
> 1 tablespoon cayenne pepper

This is an excellent gargle to avert a cold. Another version of cayenne, salt, and vinegar (page 22) is an antiflu preparation. This gargle may also be used internally. Take 1 teaspoon at a time.

To make a strong sage tea, steep a handful of the sage leaves in a pint of boiling water. Steep for twenty to thirty minutes. Strain the leaves. Combine all the other ingredients. Close bottle. Label. Shake bottle every day for about a week.

Ginger Gargle

Use this gargle for sore throat, postnasal drip, and swollen tonsils.

> 1 teaspoon ginger
> ½ cup hot water
> ½ squeezed lemon
> 1 teaspoon honey

Pour boiling water over the powdered ginger. Add lemon and honey. Either rinse out the back of the throat or gargle, making mouth motions while the gargle is held in the back of the throat. This helps alleviate sore throat pain. Alternate ginger gargle with cold pineapple juice. Between drinks, spit out mucus.

LINIMENTS

A liniment is a preparation designed for external application to the skin with a gentle friction of the hand. It is usually thicker than water, but thinner than an ointment. It is always applied as a liquid at the temperature of the body.

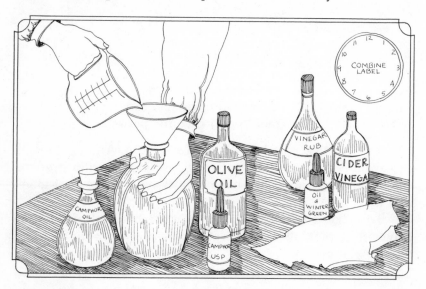

Camphorated Oil   This makes a wonderful liniment and can' be obtained from drugstores. To make your own liniment of camphor, use camphor USP.

    1   ounce camphor USP
    4   fluid ounces olive oil

Dissolve the camphor in the oil. This is an excellent aid for pain relief, sprains, bruises, rheumatic or gouty problems of the joints, and other local pains or glandular swellings. Check for skin sensitivity to camphor before full use of this liniment, however.

Vinegar Rub for Rheumatism

    1   teaspoon oil of wintergreen
    1   pint apple cider vinegar

This wintergreen vinegar is useful on inflamed rheumatic joints, stiff swollen joints, swellings, and sprains.

Soak a folded cloth in this preparation, wring out, apply to the throat, and cover with a larger, dry wool cloth or large sock. Pin it so that no air invades the area. The wintergreen will bring blood to the surface of the skin. The apple cider vinegar eases the pain and helps to release some toxins. First check for skin sensitivity to oil of wintergreen.

Pine-Cayenne Powder Vinegar Liniment

    1   pint apple cider vinegar
    6   drops oil of pine
    1   teaspoon cayenne pepper

Mix together the vinegar, oil, and cayenne powder. This can be used at body temperature, or heated and applied directly to the body, or on cloths. It is useful for strains, sprains, swollen joints, and arthritic pain. First check for skin sensitivity before using this liniment.

HERB SALT

Grind up your own herbs and use instead of common table salt.

    ⅓   total amount of recipe kelp powder
        Garlic powder
        Onion powder
        Basil
        Marjoram

Dill
Nettles
Celery seed
Papaya leaves
Comfrey leaves

Grind all ingredients into powder.

AMERICAN INDIAN ABSORBENT PAD

Dried sphagnum moss can absorb many times its own weight in water or other liquids. It was used by Indian women for menstrual periods, and for "diapers" for infants. It was also used alone, or dipped in wormwood or rue tea, garlic juice, or elderblossom tea and applied to a wound.

In drying the moss, keep it covered with cheesecloth or under the weight of a large screen to make sure it doesn't blow away.

TOOTH PREPARATIONS

Tooth Powder for Bleeding or Spongy Gums   Grind up tannin-rich herbs such as witch hazel leaves, yellow dock leaves, and bayberry leaves, and strain through a fine mesh or muslin. Use either as a tooth powder, or add boiling water, cool it off, and rinse the preparation through the mouth once or twice a day.

Sage Tooth Powder

Several handfuls sage leaves
1   handful sea salt

With a mortar and pestle, grind the leaves into the salt, and bake that in the oven until it is a green hard mass. Grind it again into a fine powder. Place it in a short but wide-mouthed ointment jar with a lid. Label. Keep the jar over the sink. Use this powder instead of toothpaste. The sage is helpful in eliminating many yellow tooth stains and has a clean taste.

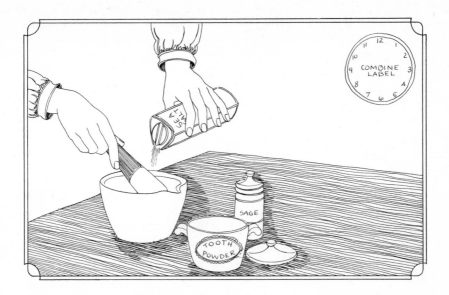

Papaya-Comfrey-Myrrh Powder

6 ounces glycerine
4 tablespoons papaya leaf powder
2 tablespoons comfrey root powder
2 tablespoons comfrey leaf powder
4 tablespoons myrrh powder (or 30 drops tincture of myrrh)
16 tablespoons (or 8 ounces) bone meal powder

Mix together the glycerine, papaya powder, and comfrey powder (all root or all leaf may be used instead of the combination). Place in tightly lidded jar, and steep for two days. Blend in the myrrh and bone meal to make a paste. Add or omit bone meal depending on the texture desired.

Marshmallow Toothbrush

Marshmallow roots cut into five-inch lengths
1 stick cinnamon
Brandy to soak

Peel and unravel the two ends of the five-inch roots and boil with a stick of cinnamon until the roots are tender. Soak in brandy. Dry in the sun or oven or warm room with circulating air. Soak in warm water to use.

The French children were once given marshmallow roots to teethe on.

Toothache   Chew cloves. If the gum is sore and there is no known cavity causing the toothache, dip the cloves in hot honey and briefly chew the cloves. For other temporary relief, place a small amount of cayenne pepper powder in the decayed tooth.

Bruised fennel plant applied externally will relieve both toothache and earache. Saturate a small wad of absorbent cotton with peppermint oil or diluted essence of peppermint, and place into decayed tooth for quick temporary relief of a toothache.

Loose Teeth   Folk legend has it that young blackberry shoots eaten in great quantities as a salad will help to fasten the teeth to the gums. See also goldenseal and myrrh.

POULTICES

A poultice is a raw or mashed herb applied directly to the body, or applied wet directly to the body, or encased in a clean cloth and then applied. Poultices are used to heal bruises, break up congestion, reduce inflammation, withdraw pus from putrid sores, soothe abrasions, or withdraw toxins from an area. They may be applied hot or cold, depending on the health need. Cold poultices (and compresses) are used to withdraw the heat from an inflamed or congested area. Use a hot poultice or compress to relax spasms and for some pains.

If the area does not respond quickly or adequately, seek the advice of a physician.

A Partial List of Effective Poultices

This list contains many everyday kitchen herbs—herbs that you will find on your grocery or refrigerator shelves, important herbs that should be found in your medicine chest, or common weeds that are found in any park, wayside, or meadow.

Arnica   Dip a cloth in arnica tincture and water, or apply arnica lotion to any *unbroken* skin bruise or sprain. Never use arnica on an open wound.

Cabbage   Wash leaf of white cabbage. Break ridges or veins. Attach to running sore. Cabbage has an affinity to pus and will draw out poisons from the body. As soon as the leaf gets hot, replace it.

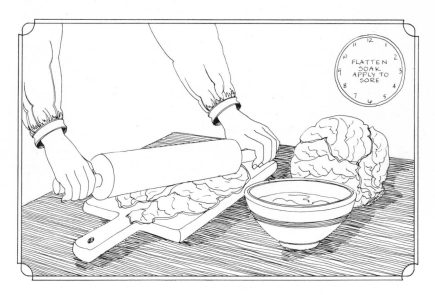

Carrot   Use raw grated carrot, or boil and mash the carrot, and crush into a pulp. Leftover juice-extractor pulp may be used for healing purposes. Apply to putrid sores. Use raw, scraped carrot pulp on chapped nipples.

Castor Oil   Apply the deodorized oil of castor oil on a cloth for inflammation, swellings, and bruises. Use hot castor oil poultices for chronic rheumatism. Keep this oil-impregnated cloth in a plastic bag and reuse whenever needed. You may heat this oil poultice with an electric heating pad whenever you wish. Castor oil is an exceptionally healing substance.

Comfrey   Apply either green mashed leaves, or slightly moistened dried green leaves, or gummy boiled roots directly to a bruise or sore, or encase in a cotton cloth and apply cloth to the body. Comfrey poultice will reduce swelling and heal skin tears and wounds.

Fig   Split open and apply hot to heal difficult sores or to bring boils to a head.

Flaxseed   Extract the healing linseed oil in the outer skin of flaxseed by boiling in water. Stir briskly with wooden spoon, and stir into either olive oil or castor oil (for hardened lumps). Dip into hot liquid, and apply hot to painful area.

Garlic   Garlic has antibacterial action and drawing power. Use it grated or boiled, added to milk and softened bread. Apply bread as a compress. It can soak out the poisons or pus.

Ginger   Simmer ginger root in water, or add powdered ginger to boiling water. Soak a folded cloth in water, and apply to relieve pain, or to bring blood to surface of congested area. Ginger may also be used for a foot soak or brief bath to reduce pain.

Marjoram   Mix equal parts of flaxseed and marjoram with a pint of boiling water. Place in clean cotton cloth, apply hot to toothache, earache, inflamed or painful area, sprains, bruises, or abscesses. Wild marjoram is stronger than sweet (pot) marjoram.

For liniment, use equal amounts of thyme, marjoram, and olive oil for backache, arthritis, sprain, charley horse, muscle soreness, bruises, rheumatism.

Sore throat: Dip folded cloth into a strong brew of marjoram and wrap around throat to relieve soreness.

Marshmallow Root releases a sweet gummy substance which can be applied tó inflamed or sore areas of the body. Make a decoction with a quarter pound of dried root and about eight glasses of water. Marshmallow tea may be added to bathwater to reduce pain.

Mustard Purchase crushed seed of mustard in the drugstore. It is an excellent rubefacient and will help reduce inflammation and congestion. It may be added to a footbath to relieve congestion in other parts of the body. To make a mustard plaster, add tepid water to make thick paste, add flour (four to one is usually sufficient). Place in folded cloth and apply to area of congestion. First apply olive oil to the skin if it is sensitive or delicate. Keep moving the plaster around the congested area. This helps break up a cold in the chest or bronchitis. (See illustration on page 269.)

Oatmeal Apply hot cooked oatmeal directly or, preferably, encased in soft cotton cloth to relieve inflammation or to help withdraw foreign objects. Use for stings and bites.

Onion Pack inflamed, bruised, injured area in roasted onion or, in an emergency, in raw onions. Onions (like carrots and turnips) have exceptional drawing power.

Plantain Plantain is a common green weed. Learn to recognize it, as it is invaluable in first-aid medicine. Apply mashed or crushed form on a cut, swollen sore, or running sore. Wrap around finger for whitlow. Attach with any clean bandage or elastic cloth. Throw away the pulp when it gets hot. Place fresh plantain on wound.

Potato Apply raw, grated potato to a bruise, sprain, black eye, boil, or carbuncle.

Rice Soak whole brown rice with a small quantity of water.

Cook briefly, or discard water and crush the rice into a paste. Apply to painful area or on wound.

Sage   Apply cool sage tea to raw abrasions or hot-leaf mash enclosed in cloth to painful area.

Salt   Heat 1 or 2 pounds of coarse salt. Wrap in pillowcase, and apply as a poultice to painful area.

Slippery Elm   The powdered bark of the slippery elm tree is one of the best healing poultices. Make into a paste with almost infinitesimal quantities of tepid water, and apply either directly to the body or contained in a clean cloth. Slippery elm powder can be added to many of the other herbs to provide an additional soothing effect. For an effective boil poultice, add slippery elm, warm water, and one cake of live yeast. For wounds, pack equal amounts of goldenseal and slippery elm powder directly to the body. Wash with sage tea, and repack with this golden "paste."

Tofu   Japanese soy bean cheese cakes will help reduce pain of inflamed areas. Squeeze out the cake, add a tablespoon or so of wheat flour, and apply to inflammation. Use this poultice alternatively with a hot, antipain ginger poultice or compress.

Turnip   Boil to soften, crush into pulp, add milk and shredded bread pulp, and apply to putrid sores, abscesses, or rheumatic area.

Vinegar   Vinegar made from either blackberries, grapes, or apples has a very healing effect on sprains, strains, sore throat, swollen glands, and aching muscles. Dip a folded cloth into such vinegar, and apply to the body. Attach with a clean bandage. For sore throat, make up a "double compress." First dip folded neck cloth into the vinegar and wring out. Apply and pin so that no air enters. Take slightly larger woolen cloth or large wool sock and pin it over the first wet, cold bandage.

Make sure no air enters. Fairly soon the throat will heat up from within, and the pain and congestion will be alleviated.

Yeast Apply yeast poultice in a cloth to a boil or painful area. Use warm milk or warm water with dried brewer's yeast, or add warm water to a live cake of yeast, or add oatmeal to a small amount of beer. Yeast may also be combined with slippery elm (an excellent combination), comfrey root or leaves, marshmallow roots, or cooked carrots.

Witch Hazel The Indians taught the pioneers the use of a decoction made from the twigs of witch hazel. The herb is exceptional in reducing minor tissue swelling on body or eyes. Distilled witch hazel is readily available in the drugstore. It is useful for sunburn, bruises, shaving cuts, eye tension, and swelling. Apply witch hazel with absorbent cotton on a small area, especially on the eyes, and with a saturated cloth for larger application.

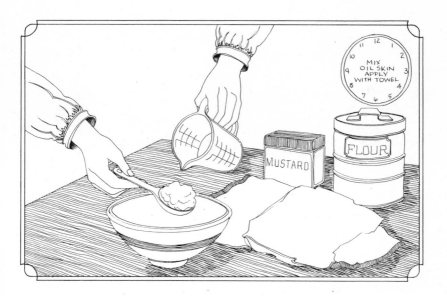

Making a mustard plaster

SECTION FOUR

RESOURCES

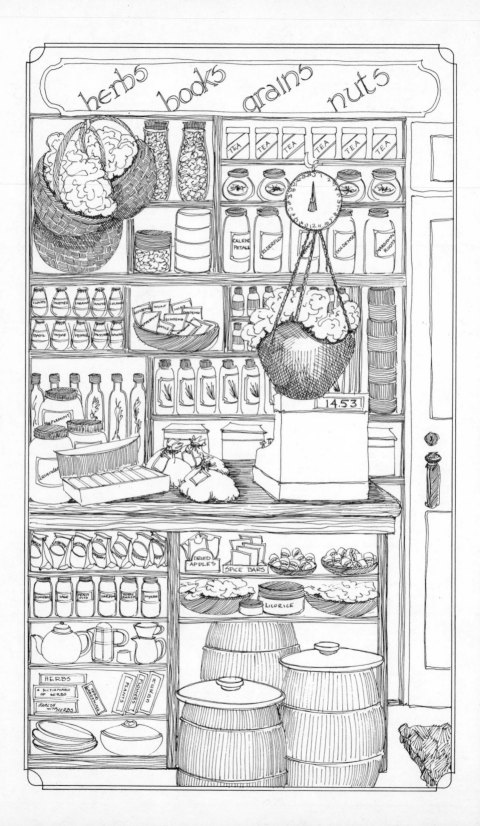

SOURCES FOR
DRIED BOTANICALS, HERB PRODUCTS,
OILS

(The starred entries are those of which the author has personal experience.)

**Aphrodisia, 28 Carmine St., N.Y., N.Y. 10014. Catalog $1.00 (worth it). Pomander sets, crystallized flowers, dried herbs, oils, hawthorn berries.

Bio-Botanica Inc, 2 Willow Park Center, Farmingdale, N.Y. 11735. The firm claims to extract with a cold, not a heat, process, thus insuring the original value in each herb. Extractions such as these (fifty or more) may help to build a herb medicine chest. However, since these are concentrates, be very careful in using them. Lobelia, pennyroyal and mistletoe are generally considered dangerous herbs, especially for new herbalists. Also note my comments on the latest research on comfrey leaf.

Black Forest Botanicals, Rt. 1, Box 34, Yuba, WI 54672.

Botanica Herbs, P.O. Box 88, Stat. N., Montreal, Canada.

Capriland's Herb Farm, Silver St., Coventry, CT 06238. Fragrances, as well as live plants and seeds, tours, herbal lunches.

**Caswell-Massey Co., Ltd., 575 Lexington Ave., N.Y., N.Y. 10017. Catalog $1.00 (collector's item each time). This is the mailing and catalog address of the oldest pharmacy in

273

the United States (Lexington Avenue and 48th Street, N.Y.C.). They mail-order excellent quality international toiletries, aromatics, herbs, soaps, and books. The Victorian catalog, which changes each season, reads like a book. The cucumber soaps and lotions are excellent.

**Culpeper the Herbalist, 21 Bruton Street, Berkeley Square, London, WIX 7DA, England. The Society of Herbalists organized this first of six imaginative herbal emporiums. They have excellent herbal products, lotions (try the almond milk), soaps, and the English edition of *Feed Your Face* (Buchman). Send a self-addressed envelope and international reply cards in exchange for air-mail stamps for personal shopping catalog.

Dandelions Unlimited, 38 W. 6th St., Covington, KY. 41011. Dandelion, slippery elm preparations.

East India Spice Co., 833 W. Trenton Ave., Morrisville, PA. 19067.

Edward's Health Center, 480 Station Rd., Quakertown, PA. 18951.

Erewhon, 33 Farnsworth St., Boston, MA. 02110. Wholesale and retail source of excellent herb and food products.

Face and Body Shop, 217 Newbury St., Boston, MA. 02116. Small store with a selection of cosmetic, culinary, aromatic, and medicinal herbs.

For Your Health, 1136 Eglington Ave. West, Toronto, M6C ZEZ, Ontario, Canada.

Geological Botany Co., 622 W. 67th St., Kansas City, MO. 64113.

GINSENG-Gae Poong Korea Ginseng, 40–15 150th Street, Flushing, N.Y. 11354.

Golden Gate Herbs, Inc., 140 Market St., San Rafael, CA. 94901.

Good Earth, 2nd Avenue & 72nd St., NY., N.Y. 10021. Large health-food store with an unusual selection of herbal teas.

Harvest Health, Inc., 1944 Eastern Ave., S.E., Grand Rapids, MI. 49507. Cosmetics, herbs, teas, health appliances.

Haussman's Pharmacy, 6th & Girard Ave., Philadelphia, PA. 19127. Tinctures, oils, coltsfoot, hawthorn, plantain, juniper juice. Catalog, 25¢.

The Herb Cottage, Washington Cathedral, Mt. St. Albans, Washington, D.C. 20016

Herb Research, Box 77212, San Francisco, CA. 94107. Medicinal herbs.

The Herb Store, P.O. Box 5756, Sherman Oaks, CA. 91403.

Herb's Herbs, P.O. Box 577, New Canaan, CT. 06840. Spices, herbal footbaths, skin ointments.

The Herb House, P.O. Box 308, Beaumont, CA. 92223.

Herbs & Spices by Panacea, 323 Third Avenue, N.Y., N.Y. 10010.

Herbs of Mexico, 3859 Whittier Blvd., Los Angeles, CA. 90023. Herbs from all over the world.

Hershey Estates, Hershey, PA. 17033. Soaps, cosmetics, cocoa butter.

Indiana Botanic Gardens, Inc., Hammond, IN. 46325. Gums, oils, resins, herb preparations.

Kalustyan Orient Export Trading Corp., 123 Lexington Ave., N.Y., N.Y. 10016. Herbs, spices, grains.

Kiehl Pharmacy, 109 Third Ave., N.Y., N.Y. 10003. No catalog. Reliable source of fragrances, dried herbs, Kiehl products, including valerian discotes, purified lanolin liquid, neutral and colored henna with chamomile.

Kramer's Health-Food Store, 29 East Adams St., Chicago, IL. 60603.

Lady Bug Natural Products, P.O. Box 873, Shelly, MN. 56581.

*⁎*Larsen's Country Herb Shop, Box 253, Orem, UT. 84057. Toll free 1-800-453-2400; Utah 1-800-662-2500. Excellent mail-order source of comfrey and other ointments, tinctures, live aloe plants, capsules, and packaged herbs. This is also called Nature's Herb, but is not the one in San Francisco.

Lekvar by the Barrel (or Roth's), 1577 First Ave., N.Y., N.Y. 10028. Father Kneipp pure juice, dried herbs, spices, kitchen gadgets, etc.

Lewiston Health-Food Center, 861 Main, Lewiston, ID. 83501.

Lhasa Karnack Herb Co., 2482 Telegraph Ave., Berkeley, CA. 94704. Many smoking and other blends.

Magus, P.O. Box 254, Cedar Grove, N.J. 07009. A wholesale and mail-order firm who say many of the herbs and spices they sell are "organic and wild, having been picked along the Appalachian Trail." Also, some books, water distiller, filter and organic cotton bags for herb teas, sachets, bouquet garni.

*⁎*Meadowbrook Herb Farm, Route 138, Wyoming, R.I. 02898. Catalog 50¢. Organic farm with excellent dried herbs available in many health-food stores. They carry cosmetics from West Germany (famed Dr. R. Hauschka line), herbs, spices.

Dr. Michael's Herb Products, 5109 North Western Ave., Chicago, IL. 60625.

Mission Garden Products, 4041 First St., Riverside, CA. 92501. Herb foods, seasonings, spices, sauces, etc.

Steve Mohorko Co., 16803 Ceres Ave., Fontana, CA. 92335. Herbs, seeds, spices.

Murchie's, 1008 Robson St., Vancouver, 105, B.C., Canada. Teas, coffees, spices.

*⁎*D. Napier & Sons, 17 Bristo Place, Edinburgh, EHI, Scotland.

The first herbalist, Napier, organized this pharmacy in 1860, and it is the oldest family herb emporium in Scotland. There is a marvelous slippery elm soap, and many other family products and creams. They do mail-order. Send a self-addressed envelope and international reply cards to pay for air-mail postage. I visited with Mr. Napier in Scotland. The place is unique.

Natural Development Co., Box 215, Bainbridge, PA. 17502. Some culinary herbs, edible lipsticks, sprouting seeds, soil testers.

Nature's Herbs, Inc. (See Larsen's.)

Nature's Herb Company, 281 Ellis Street, San Francisco, CA. 94102. Herbs for medical use, potpourri, and essential oils.

Nature's Own, Box 311M, East Granby, CT. 06026. Catalog 25¢.

McNulty's Tea & Coffee Co., Inc. 109 Christopher St., N.Y., N.Y. 10014.

Nelson's Natural Foods, 1558 Central Park Ave., Yonkers, N.Y. 10710.

*⁎*Northwestern Co., 217 North Broadway, Milwaukee, WI. 53202. Spices, nuts, teas, Melior coffee infuser (excellent for herbal teas), mortar and pestles.

Ohio Comfrey Growers, Rt. 1, Box 289A, Millport, OH. 43046. Comfrey.

Organic Farm and Garden Center, 767 Lincoln Ave., San Rafael, CA. 94901. Organic fertilizer and supplies.

Organic Foods & Gardens, 2655 Commerce Way, Los Angeles, CA. 90040.

Organic Notions, 165 Page St., San Francisco, CA. 94102. Organic cosmetics, soaps.

Organics, 915 24th Ave., East, Tuscaloosa, AL. 35401. Organic pesticides. $1-Sampler kit. Free information.

Paprikas Weiss, Importers, 1546 Second Ave., N.Y., N.Y. 10028. Dried culinary herbs and spices, honey, gourmet gadgets galore. Herbs sold in apothecary jars. Famed source.

Patton Vegetarian Products, 1712 E. 22nd St., Los Angeles, CA. 90058. Herb teas, dressings, salt, shampoos.

S. B. Penick & Co., 100 Church St., N.Y., N.Y. 10007. Distributors of bulk imported botanicals. World famous. Distributed by Wunderlich-Diez.

**Penn Herb Co., 603 N. 2nd St., Philadelphia, PA. 19123. Excellent dried herbal source and distributor of renowned Olbas herbal lotion and oil, and books.

The Redwood City Seed Co., P.O. Box 361, Redwood City, CA. 94064. Excellent source of rare nuts, berries, and herbs.

**Otto Richter & Sons, Ltd., Locust Hill, Ontario, Canada. Excellent and varied selection of rare herbs.

Rocky Hollow Herb Farm, Lake Wallkill Road, Sussex, N.J. 07461. Well-presented dried herb packages sold through many health-food stores.

H. Roth & Son (See Lekvar by the Barrel.)

Rolly's Health-Food Store, 634 Yonge St., Toronto, Ontario, Canada. Medicinal herbs and health foods.

Frederic Sadler, Inc., Box 323, Fort Washington, PA. 19034. Seeds for sprouting, and the famed Beale's clay sprouter.

Schapira Coffee Co., 117 W. 10th St., N.Y., N.Y. 10011. Rare teas, some herbs.

**Serenity, 310 E. 72nd St., N.Y., N.Y. 10021.

A. Shamrock, P.O. Box 40900, San Francisco, CA. 94110. Herb brokers, mail-order herbs.

The Soap Box at Truc, 40 Brattle St., Cambridge, MA. 02138. Natural toiletries, oils, perfume burner.

The Soap Opera, 312 State St., Madison, WI. 53703. Mixed selection of biodegradable cosmetics, bath, oil, toiletry products.

**Star Herb Co., 352 Miller Ave., Mill Valley, CA. 94941. Importers and distributers of botanicals and ginseng.

Stillridge Herb Farm, 10370 Rt. 99, Woodstock, MD. 21163. Catalog 35¢ (refundable with order). Eighteenth-century potpourri and pomander kits.

Tatra Herb Co., 222 Grove St., Morrisville, PA. 19067.

Vermont Country Store, Weston, VT. 05161. Condiments, spices, herbs, grains. Real horehound candy.

**Weleda, 30 S. Main St., Spring Valley, N.Y. 10977. Excellent bath, toiletry, medical preparations, lotions, ointments. Famed hayflower extract from Europe, rosemary bath lotion. Outlet for top European products.

Wide World of Herbs, Ltd., 11 St. Catherine St. East, Montreal, 129, Canada. Fairly inexpensive resource.

World Health Products, Broadway & 84th St., N.Y., N.Y. 10024. Health-food store with unusual selection of herbal teas and products.

Wunderlich-Dietz Corp., State Highway 17, Hasbrouck Heights, N.J. 07604. Celandine tincture used as panacea herb by many Europeans, other herbal preparations, tinctures, bath products. U.S.A. sales rep for S. B. Penick & Co. (1050 Wall St. West, Lyndhurst, N.J. 07071).

LIVE PLANT AND SEED SOURCES

Applewood Seed Co., 833 Parfet St., Lakewood, CO. 80215. A stress here on herb seeds that existed in Shakespeare's era.

Vernon Barnes & Sons Nursery, P.O. Box 250, McMinnville,

TN. 37110. Many medicinal trees, fruit trees, vines, flowers, ground covers, berries, evergreens.

Blackthorne Gardens, 48 Quincy St., Holbrook, MA. 02343. Rhubarb (a dye), raspberries, horseradish, garlic.

BlueRidge Ginseng, McDonald, TN. 37353. Ginseng seed.

Borchelt Herb Gardens, 474 Carriage Shop Rd., East Falmouth, MA. 02536. Plants, seeds, teas, pomander, garden tours.

Bunting's Nurseries, Selbyville, DEL. 19975. Berries, evergreens, flowers, fruits, nuts.

Burgess Seed and Plant Co., Galesberg, MI. 49053. Berries and sprouting supplies.

W. Atlee Burpee Co., 6350 Rutland, Riverside, CA. 92502. Seeds, books, starter sets, plant stands, greenhouses.

Caplilands, Coventry, CT. 06238 Eighteenth-century farmhouse, herbal garden shop. Tours and herb luncheons served.

Carroll Gardens, P.O. Box 310, East Main St., Westminster, MD. 21157. Lady mantle, elecampane, chamomile, camphor tree, excellent perennials and herbs, comfrey, fennel, catmint, horehound, angelica.

Casa Yerba, Star Rt. 2, Box 21, Day's Creek, OR. 97429. Catalog 50¢. Excellent variety of plants and seeds, good descriptions, pollen, books.

Cedarbrook Herb Farm, Rt. 1, Box 1047, Sequim, WA. 98382. No mail orders.

Clearwater Farms, Des Arc, MO. 63636. Ginseng seed.

Comstock, Ferre & Co., 263 Main Street, Wethersfield, CT. 06109. No mail orders. Medicine, history, design, flavoring.

Conley's Garden Center, Boothbay Harbor, ME. 04583. Wildflowers, ferns, boneset.

Country Herbs, 3 Maple St., Stockbridge, MA. 01262. Plant list 25¢. Yarn sample 50¢. 130 varieties organically grown medicinal, culinary, aromatic, and dye plants.

DeGiorgi Company, Inc., Council Bluffs, IA. 51501. Catalog 35¢. Chamomile, cinnamon vine.

The Dutch Mill Herb Farm, Rt. 2, Box 190, Forest Grove, OR. 97116. Monthly newsletter. Sample 15¢.

Farmer Seed & Nursery Co., Faribault, MN. 55021. Elderberries, cranberry.

Ferndale Nursery & Greenhouse, P.O. Box 218, Askov, MN. 55704. Wild ginger, blue cohosh.

Ferry-Morse Seed Co., Box 200, Fulton, KY. 42041. Herbs, citrus fruits, flower seeds.

Henry Field Seed & Nursery Co., Shenandoah, IA. 51602. Household, culinary herbs.

Fox Hill Farm, Box 1, Parma, MI. 49269. Catalog 50¢. Good brochure, dictionary, and classification of herb use.

Andrew Gallant, Rt. 2, Albion, PA. 16401. Garlic seed.

The Gardener's Cupboard, Box 4061-12P, Terre Haute, IN. 47804. Aloe vera plants.

Gardens of the Blue Ridge, Ashford, N.C. 28603. Excellent source of wildflowers, garden plants, sweet flag, joe pye, oswego.

Gilberties Herb Garden, Sylvan Avenue, Westport, CT. 06860. Two hundred varieties of herb plants.

M. Girvan, Stanhope, IA. 50246. Catalog 25¢. Jewelweed seeds (juice of stem poison ivy aid).

Green Herb Gardens, Greene, R.I. 02827. Excellent source of herb seeds, including pot marigold (calendula).

Gurney Seed & Nursery Co., Yankton, S.D. 57078. Culinary herbs.

Halcyon Gardens, Gibsonia, PA. 15044. By appointment. One hundred varieties culinary, medical, fragrant herbs.

Joseph Harris Co., Moreton Farm, Rochester, N.Y. 14624. Culinary herbs.

Heine's Wausau Farms, Rt. 3, Wausau, WI. 54401.

Hemlock Hill Herb Farm, Litchfield, CT. 06759. Catalog 50¢. Perennial herbs.

The Herb Farm, Barnard Rd., Granville, MA. 01034.

Herbs "n" Honey Nursery, Rt. 2, Box 205, Monmouth, OR. 97361. Family herb farm, wide variety of organic herb plants, dried herbs.

Hi Mountain Farm, Seligman, MO. 65745. Wild flowers from the Ozark Mountains.

Hickory Hollow, Rt. 1, Box 52, Peterstown, W. VA. 24963.

Hilltop Herb Farm, Box 866, Cleveland, TX. 77327. Plants, herb vinegars, herb salts, potpourri kits, pomander ball kits, canning products.

Howe Hill Herbs, Camden, ME. 04843. Catalog 50¢.

J. H. Hudson, Seedsman, P.O. Box 1058, Redwood City, CA. 94064. Terrific source of medicinal and other herb seeds: calendula, valerian, chamomile, etc.

International Growers Exchange, Box 397, Farmington, MI. 48021. Rare plants from all over the world.

International House, 75 W. Island Ave., Minneapolis, MN. 55401. Exotic plants and plant accessories.

Le Jardin du Gourmet, Box 245, Ramsey, N.J. 07446. Excellent herbs, spices, and seeds.

Jewel Tea Co., Inc., 1955 W. North Avenue, Melrose Park, IL. 60160. Teas and general merchandise.

Johnny's Selected Seeds, Albion, ME. 04910. Organic seeds for luffa sponge, white clover, burdock.

Joseph Kern Rose Nursery, Box 33, Mentor, OH. 44060.

Kitazawa Seed Co., 356 W. Taylor St., San Jose, CA. 95110. Japanese and Chinese vegetable seeds, mustards, and healing Japanese radish—daikon.

Kitchawan Plant Shop, Kitchawan Research Station of Brooklyn Botanic Garden, Route 134, Ossining, N.Y. 10562 (bt. Route 100 and Taconic Parkway).

Frank Lemaster & Co., Rt. 1, Londonderry, OH. 45647.

Leodar Nurseries, 7206 Belvedere Rd., West Palm Beach, FLA. 33406

Leslie's Wildflower Nursery, 30 Summer Street, Methuen, MA. 01844. Wildflowers, ferns, boneset, wild ginger, vervain, arnica, cinquefoil.

Logee's Greenhouses, 55 North St., Danielson, CT. 06239. Catalog 50¢. Excellent source of culinary herbs.

Mail Box Seeds, Shirley Morgan, 2042 Encinal Ave., Alameda, CA. 94501. Excellent source of seeds.

McFarland House Garden Shop & Greenhouses, 5923 Exchange St., McFarland, WI. 53558. Many herbs.

Merry Gardens, Camden, ME. 04843. Excellent source of culinary, some medicinal herbs.

Midwest Wildflowers, Box 64, Rockton, IL. 61072. Many medicinal wildflowers and others.

Miller Nurseries, Inc., Canandaigua, N.Y. 14424.

Mitchell's Herb & Vegetable Acre, 9819 Lake June Rd., Dallas TX. 75217. Organic herbs. No shipping.

Nichols Garden Nursery, 1190 North Pacific Highway, Albany, ORE. 97321. Hard-to-get plants, herbs, peppermint oil from the Oregon peppermint fields, seeds.

Ohio Comfrey Growers, Rt. 1, Box 289A, Millersport, OH. 43046. Comfrey roots.

Olds Seed Co., Box 1068, Madison, WI. 53701. Seeds, culinary herbs, starter garden.

Orchid Gardens, Rt. 1, Grand Rapids, MN. 55744. Some wildflowers.

George W. Park Seed Co., P.O. Box 31, Greenwood, S.C. 29646. Starter herb sets, culinary seeds, plant stands.

Theodore Payne Foundation, 10459 Turford St., Sun Valley, CA. 91352. California wildflowers and plants.

Pine Hills Herb Farm, P.O. Box 144, Roswell, GA. 30075.

Plant Oddities, Box 127, Basking Ridge, N.J. 07926. Unusual nursery stock.

Putney Nursery, Inc., Box 13, Putney, VT. 05346. Wildflowers, some medicinal flowers.

The Ramson Seed Co., Campbell, Devon Lane, Newport Beach, CA. 92660. Berries, flowers, seeds, trees.

Otto Richter & Sons, Ltd., Box 26A, Goodwood, Ontario, Canada LOCIAO. Catalog 50¢. Three hundred varieties of herb seeds. Excellent and interesting catalog.

Clyde Robin, P.O. Box 2091, Castro Valley, CA. 94546. Catalog, $1.00. Interesting, rare wildflower plants and seeds. Good catalog.

Rutland of Kentucky, Rt. 1, Box 17, Maysville, KY. 41506. Catalog $1.50 (refundable). Retail and contract herb specialists.

Savage Farm Nursery, Box 125, McMinnville, TN. 37110.

R. H. Shumway, Seedsman, P. O. Box 777, Rockford, IL. 61101.

Smirz's Herb Nursery, 5573 Northridge, Rt. 20, Madison, OH. 44057. Interesting choices and plants.

Snow Line Farm, 11846 Fremont, Yucaipa, CA. 92399.

Sperka's Woodland Acres Nursery, Crivitz, WI. 54114. Hardy wildflowers and ferns. Celandine.

Stoke's Seeds, Inc., Box 548, Buffalo, N.Y. 14240. Lots of herbs. Check each page of the catalog.

Sunnybrook Farms Nursery, 9448 Mayfield Rd., Chesterland, OH. 44026. Catalog 50¢ (deductible).

Suttons Seeds Ltd., The Royal Seed Establishment, London Rd., Earley, Reading, Berkshire, England. Send international reply cards for catalog. Good culinary seeds. Eucalyptus.

Taylor's Herb Gardens, Inc., 1535 Lone Oak Road, Vista, CA. 92083. Free catalog. Two hundred live medicinal, culinary, and aromatic herb plants. Excellent source, open since 1947.

Thomasville Nurseries, Inc., Thomasville, GA. 31792. Specialty flowers and shrubs.

Thompson & Morgan, 401 Kennedy Blvd., Somerdale, N.J. 08083. English firm with American outlet. Some medicinal, many culinary seeds.

Three Laurels, Rt. 3m, Marshall, N.C. 28753. Wildflower and garden plants, some medicinal herbs, witch hazel, goldenseal, berries.

Tillotson's Roses, 802 Brown's Valley Rd., Watsonville, CA. 95076. Rose hips, rosewater, and rock rose, good medicine. Rose buds, important aromatics.

The Tool Shed Herb Farm, Turkey Hill Road, Salem Center, Burdy's Station, N.Y. 10570. Catalog 25¢. Small herb farm with excellent plants.

Tropical Paradise Greenhouse, 8825 W. 79th St., Overland Park, KS. 66204. Wildflower and hothouse plants.

Moses J. Troyer, Lone Organic Farm, Rt. 1, Box 58, Millersburg, IN. 46543. Small farm. Source of bottled Dr. Bach Rescue Remedy.

Vick's Wildgardens, Inc., Box 115, Gladwyne, PA. 19035.

Martin Viette Nurseries, East Norwich, N.Y. 11732. Source English lavender.

Vita Green Farms, P.O. Box 878, Vista, CA. 92083. Organic seeds and vegetables.

Wells Sweep Herb Farm, 451 Mt. Bethel Rd., Port Murray, N.J. 07865. Cyrus Hyde's reconstruction. Herb plants, seeds, dried flowers, lecture tours by appointment.

Mrs. M. C. White, 67616 Hacienda Drive, Desert Hot Springs, CA. 92240. Aloe vera, citrus fruits, vegetables.

White Mountain Farm, Litchfield, CT. 06759. Mail source of excellent English lavender (*Lavandula augustifolia* formerly *vera.*)

The Wild Garden, P.O. Box 487, Bothell, WA. 98011.

Woodstream Nursery, Box 510, Jackson, N.J. 08527. Excellent wildflower, medical herb source.

World Organic, P.O. Box 8207, Fountain Valley, CA. 92700. Comfrey.

Yankee Peddler Herb Farm, Rt. 4, Box 76, Hwy. 36N, Brenham, TX. 77833. Catalog $1.00 (refundable). Arnica, chia, mullein, shepherd's purse, fenugreek, jewelweed, marshmallow, borage, etc.

The Yarb Patch, 3726 Thomasville Rd., Tallahassee, FL. 32303.

SOCIETIES

American Horticulture Society
Mt. Vernon, VA. 22121

New York Horticulture Society
128 West 58th Street, New York, N.Y. 10019

New York Botanical Garden
Bronx, New York 10458

The Herb Society (of England)
Dr. M. Stuart, Director
34 Boscobel Pl.
London, S.W. 1

They publish an excellent magazine: the *Herbal Review*. Send international reply card to cover mailing reply. Overseas membership is £9 per year (ask bank for dollar value).

National Food Association
P.O. Box 210
Atlanta, Texas 75551

One of the first organizations in the United States to concern itself with organic farming and food resources. They have state chapters and conferences.

National Health Federation
212 Foothill Blvd.
Monrovia, CA. 91016

National Foundation for the Prevention of Oral Disease
P.O. Box 14963
Phoenix, Arizona 85063

The Huxley Institute
1209 California Road
Eastchester, N.Y. 10709

One of the active Huxley branches. They keep tabs on nutrition-minded physicians.

East-West Foundation
359 Boylston St.
Boston, MA. 02116

Oriental Medicine, theory. Several chapters around the country.

Herb Trade Association
P.O. Box 648
Boulder, CO. 80306

Newsletter and an auxiliary membership ($10.00) as a Friend of Herbs.

The Herb Society of America
300 Massachusetts Avenue
Boston, MA. 02115

This is a membership by sponsorship and election. The main thrust of this Society is toward herb gardening for fragrant, culinary, and decorative uses. They publish many informative pamphlets, and an annual, *The Herbalist*, which can be purchased by subscription.

Application for membership should be sent to the Chairman of the Membership Committee. There are fifteen units of the Society scattered all over the United States.

Note: The organization is not interested in medicinal use of herbs except in the historical use in the past.

Canadian Herbalists Association
43500 Chillwalk Mt. Rd.
Sardis, B.C.,
Canada

MAGAZINES WITH HEALTH AND HERBAL INFORMATION

Mother Earth News
P.O. Box 70
Hendersonville, N.C. 28739

Excellent alternative living and homesteading magazine.

The Health Quarterly
36 Grove Street
New Canaan, CT. 06840

Buy in health-food stores; no subscriptions at this time. At only 25¢ the best buy in the country.

The Herbalist
P.O. Box 53
Spanish Fork, Utah 84660

All about herbs for medicine, cooking, cosmetics, aromatics. An excellent monthly.

Let's Live
444 North Larchmont Blvd.
Los Angeles, CA. 90004

Nutrition and health magazine.

Organic Gardening and Farming
Emmaus, PA. 18048.

The first magazine with organic information.

Prevention
Emmaus, PA. 18048

Geared to the prevention of disease. Many herbal articles.

International College of Applied Nutrition
La Habra, CA. 90631

An organization with excellent, up-to-date nutritional bulletins and conference cassettes.

The Herb Quarterly
Box 576
Wilmington, VT 05363

BOOKS AND BOOKSTORES

The Heritage Bookstore, Inc.
P.O. Box 444
Virginia Beach, VA. 23458

Mail order books and herbal items, particularly those advised by Edgar Cayce.

Homeopathic Bookstore
Wehawken Book Co.
5104 Wehawken Road
Washington, D.C. 20016

Aurora Books
P.O. Box 358
Denver, CO 80201

Hard-to-find health books in every category. Send for catalog.

Penn Herb Company
Caswell-Massey Pharmacy
Country Herb Shop
(See herb source listing for these three.)

A Guide to Medicinal Plants of Appalachia
Agricultural Handbook #400
Government Printing Office
Washington, D.C. 10402 $3.85

The government prints many bulletins and books of interest to herbal gardeners. This is illustrated, and an excellent overview of Appalachian use of herbs.

The Herb House
P.O. Box 308
Beaumont, CA. 92223

If you read Spanish, this may interest you. They carry the definitive Spanish works *Las Plantas Medicinales de México*.

Native Michigan Herbs
Herb Society of America
Southern Michigan Unit

Herbs used by Indians for medicine and food.

ASI Medical Booklist
127 Madison Avenue
New York, NY 10016

A health and herb book catalog.

Yes! Bookshop
1035 31st Street, N.W.
Washington, D.C. 20007

Books on health, healing, herbs, and medicine. Catalog 50¢

Dr. Edward Bach Centre
Mount Vernon, Sotwell, Wallingford
Great Britain OX10 OP2

All six books on the Bach Flower Remedies. Also a newsletter.

Samuel Weiser, Inc.
740 Broadway
New York, N.Y. 10003

Health books from all over the world. Mail orders accepted.

HERB IDENTIFICATION

Field Guide to Wildflowers
Peterson and McKinney

Hard- and soft-cover editions. The flowers are arranged by color. This makes random field identification simple and productive. A must for all season identification.

Master Herbalist Game
BiWorld Publishers
P.O. Box 62
Provo, UT 84601

A game testing your knowledge of herbs and herbal remedies.

"Edible and Poisonous Plants of
  • Eastern States"
  • Western States"
Lake Oswego, OR. 97034

Identification cards the size of playing cards.

Survival Playing Cards
Above address or
Rt. 2, Box 508
Hood River, OR. 97031

Wall Charts

New York Botanical Garden
Bronx, N.Y. 10458

Free catalog. The Botanical Garden has an excellent gift and mail-order department. They import the most beautiful color charts I have ever seen. Each chart is breathtaking and quite useful. They don't have a chart of medicinal plants, but rather show plants in native habitat. The Garden also sells striking color prints, including a series from *Hortus Eystettensis*, 1613.

Herbal Holding Co.,
P.O. Box 5854,
Sherman Oaks, CA. 91413.

Herbal Remedy Chart, Culinary Herb Chart, Dial "N" Herb Wheel, Tibetan Corrective Eyechart.
But don't purchase the mint Bidi cigarettes—toxic plant included.

SCHOOL

California School of Herbal Studies
P.O. Box 350
Guerneville, CA 95446

Walks, retreats, classes, workshops.

CLAY RESOURCES

The Three Sheaves Co.
16 Hudson Street
New York, N.Y. 10013

French and other clay products for internal and external healing.

Weleda
841 South Main Street
Spring Valley, N.Y. 10977
  Retail Pharmacy:
Hungry Hollow Road and Rt. 45
Spring Valley, N.Y. 10977

Luvos #1 and #2 for internal and external healing purposes. Firm carries herbal baths including hayflower and rosemary.

Jordan clay.

You might want to check local resource for this clay, as you might want to pick it up to save shipping. Pottery supply houses keep this neutral clay in stock.

HOMEOPATHIC PHARMACIES

Boericke and Tafel
1011 Arch Street
Philadelphia, PA. 19107

Excellent calendula products, home homeopathic kit, other needs. Very old and respected pharmacy.

Nelson's Pharmacy
73 Duke Street
Grosvenor Square
London, WIM 6 BY,
England

This is one of the most dignified and oldest homeopathic pharmacies in the world, and they send materials all over the world. I had the pleasure of a long visit to the central pharmacy and an extended investigation of the factory. They have a home kit and many herbal products in homeopathic form. They also carry the Rescue Remedy ointment, and other Bach flower remedies. Send an International Reply Card for information.

Bio-Natural Health Aids, Distributors
Box 186
Scarborough, N.Y. 10510

Mail-order firm distributing directly from homeopathic man-
ufacturers in London and Germany. Tinctures, tissue salts,
homeopathic medicines, toothpaste, books, pure herbal juices.
(Also see book list.)

Dr. Edward Bach Flower Remedies

See Books and Bookstores.

Hahn & Hahn Homeopathic Pharmacy
324 W. Saratoga Street
Baltimore, MD. 21201

Luyties Phrmacal Co.
4200 Laclede Ave.
St. Louis, MO. 63108

Erhart and Karl
17 North Wabash Ave.
Chicago, IL. 60602

Kiehl's Pharmacy
109 3rd Ave.
New York, N.Y. 10003

No mail order. Old, excellent source of herbs, oils and
homeopathic materials.

OLD PHARMACEUTICAL PREPARATIONS

Eli Lilly and Co.
740 South Alabama St.
Indianapolis, IN. 46206

These are the old standards and should still be in your
pharmacist's daily stock. Tinctures of: valerian, gentian,

myrrh, benzoin, arnica; camphor liniment, wild cherry extract; licorice (glycyrrhiza) fluid extract.

MISCELLANEOUS RESOURCES

Gelatin Capsules

Pure Planet
Box 675-B
Tempe, AZ. 85281

Paul Larsen's Nature's Herb
Box 253
Orem, UT. 84057 (See Herb Resources List.)

Wine

Bully Hill Wine Co.
Hammondsport, N.Y. 14840

This wine, which is distributed throughout the country, is made by one family and is aged in oak barrels. No adulterants are used.

Old Bottles

Bottles Unlimited
245 East 78th Street
New York, N.Y. 10021
628-8769

New Bottles that Look Old

Bathsheba's Bottle Barn
P.O. Box 1776
Milleville, N.J. 08332

Aloe

Aloe Products
10422 Telephone Road
Houston, TX. 77034

Swiss Herbal Remedies, Ltd.
790 Supertest Road
Downsview, Ontario M352M5
Canada

Herbal Wine Vinegar

American Industries Corp.
814 Montgomery Street
San Francisco, CA. 94133

Farming Teacher

Carla Emory
Box 1
Kendrick, ID. 83537

Carla brings in professional farmers from all over the country to teach in her summer sessions right on her own farm. All the things your farming grandfather could have taught you, but you forgot to ask!

Herbal Pet Products

Harmony Hill
433 Beaumont Blvd.
Pacifica, CA. 94044
Catalog $1.

Flea collars and other herbal products. Herbs can be just as successful for pets as they are with your family.

Research People, Inc.
So. Rt. Box 12
Lavina, MT. 59046

Flea collars for dogs and cats made of pennyroyal and eucalyptus.

Wildflower Designs for Needlepoint

February 1977 issue of *Better Homes and Gardens* contains eight tear-out pages of full-size originals.

Wildflower Crewel Kits

Better Homes and Gardens
Box 374
Des Moines, IA. 50336

Herbal Design Needlepoint

New York Unit
Herb Society of America
P.O. Box 182
Golden's Bridge, N.Y. 10526

Groups of several designs.

Herb Garden Samplers, Herbal Tiles

Western Pennsylvania Unit
Herb Society of America
Miss Nancy Hood
1 Le Moyne Ave. Ext.
Washington, PA. 15301

Wildflower Notepaper

National Wildlife Federation
1412 Sixteenth St., N.W.
Washington, D.C. 20036

New York Botanical Garden Gift Catalog
Bronx, N.Y. 10458

Herb Design Canvas Apron

"Parsley, Sage, Rosemary, and Thyme"
New York Unit
Herb Society of America
392 Harris Road
Bedford Hills, N.Y. 10507

Traveling Sprout Bag

Rainbow Designs
Box 1057
Columbia, CA. 95310

Handmade cotton bag for raising sprouts at home, but particularly while traveling.

Herbal Design Stained Glass

Metropolitan Museum of Art
82nd Street at Fifth Avenue
New York, N.Y. 10028
Gift catalog.

Calico, Sage, and Thyme
115 Clay
Bowling Green, OH. 43402
(15¢ stamp)

Herbal Juices

Schoenenberger Fresh Herbal Juices. Natural, pure cellular juices of fresh plants, cultivated without insecticides, biocides, or sprays of any kind, and to which no water has been added. The following juices are available from health food stores or distributor: black radish, borage, chamomile, celery, dandelion, hawthorn, horsetail, melissa (balm), nettle, paprika, parsley, pumpkin, rosemary, thyme, valerian, watercress, wormwood, yarrow.

Bio-Nutritional Products,
P.O. Box 389,
Harrison, N.Y. 10528

This distributor, formerly Sea & Earth in New York City, has many valuable biological and nutritional products.

Chia Bird Sprouter
Norma
1500 S. Surf Rd. #17
Hollywood, FL. 33019

Chia seeds are tender in salads or soups or eaten as sprouts. They contain many minerals and vitamins, and are said to be slightly laxative. They have a reputation gleaned through American Indian use, and are said to be exceptionally energizing.

The seeds are very, very small and are normally hard to sprout. This sprouter works by creating a feathery effect on the bird. The sprouts are cut off as needed. Send $9.30 for bird sprouter and handling; an additional dollar for extra seeds.

Tonic

Chico-San
P.O. Box 10004
Chico, CA. 95926

Bainiku ekisu—a Japanese tonic made from Japanese green plums. Add a few drops to your herbal tea.

Tekka—high-mineral flavoring with ginger, lotus, and burdock root. Very cleansing for the system and digestive aid.

FILMS ABOUT HERBAL MEDICINE

Appalshop Films,
Box 743,
Whiteburg, KY. 41858.
Send for a catalog.

This is a unique, nonprofit cooperative of young Appalachian people devoted to showing the traditions of doctoring, birthing, and living, as well as crafts. Three films of interest:

"Catfish: Man of the Woods," twenty-seven minutes, color, sale/$300, rental/$25. The story of Clarence Gray, a fifth-generation folk medicine practitioner, as he reads his mail orders for various herbs, hunts through the woods for ginseng and angelica, handles a black snake, and talks, talks, talks about his mountain philosophy.

"Nature's Way," twenty-two minutes, color, sale/$250, rental/$25. A quintette of mountain people, and the practice of folk medicine: a fast-talking, old-fashioned "medicine man"; Etta Banks, an old mountain woman making her home salve of balm of gilead and mutton and lard; a black farming couple talking of home nostrums and ginger "stir" with corn liquor, and their cure for the seven-year-itch; Kern Kiser, who shows his remedies with red raspberry, slippery elm bark, and all of the clovers—red, white, and purple; and, my favorite sequence, Lena Stephens, a plain, hard-working, and capable midwife as she gently eases a young mountain girl in her birth of twin girls.

"Mountain Farmer" nine minutes, black and white, sale/$100, rental/$10. Shows wizened Lee Banks coaxing vegetables and potatoes from the ground. "I never bought no meat nor lard for fifty years."

A PARTIAL LIST OF SOME OLD RESTORED HERBAL GARDENS

National Herb Gardens
U.S. National Arboretum
Washington, D.C.

A $250,000 bicentennial gift to the nation from the Herb Society of America.

The Robison York State Garden
Cornell University
Ithaca, N.Y.

Designed as a living reference library for herb study with 800 species of herbs, including those linked to ancient China, Babylonia, India, Greece, Rome, medieval Europe, and Indians and colonists of upstate New York.

Restored gardens
Williamsburg, Virginia
Ten herbs in packet from
Craft House
Williamsburg, VA 23185

Van Cortlandt Manor at Croton-on-Hudson
Tarrytown, N.Y. 10591

Old herbs from earlier times are planted, and costumed hostesses present information and recipes with ancient cookware.

Western Reserve Herb Garden
Garden Center of Greater Cleveland
11030 East Boulevard
Cleveland, OH 44106

Bartow-Pell Mansion Museum and Garden
Pelham Bay Park, N.Y. 10464
Restored and maintained by International Garden Club, Inc.

The Herb Garden
The New York Botanical Garden
Bronx, N.Y. 10458

Designed and maintained by the New York Unit of the Herb Society of America.

Garden of Exploration
Arkansas School for the Blind
(Medical garden included.)

Herb Garden of the Brooklyn Botanical Garden
Eastern Parkway
Brooklyn, N.Y.

17th-Century Garden
Quincy Homestead
Hancock Street and Butler Road
Quincy, MA. 02169

18th-century Garden
Ironmaster's House
Old Saugus Ironworks
Saugus, ME.

Hortulus Herb Garden
National Cathedral
Washington, D.C.

Colonial Herb Garden
The American Museum in Britain
Claverton Manor, Bath
England

INDEX

305